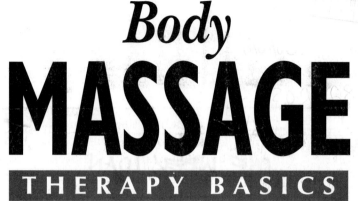

Body MASSAGE
THERAPY BASICS

Mo Rosser

Hodder & Stoughton

A MEMBER OF THE HODDER HEADLINE GROUP

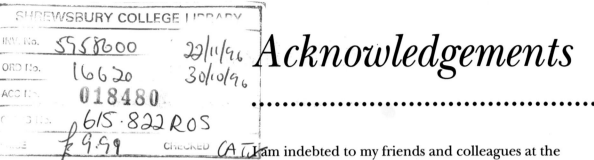
Acknowledgements

....

I am indebted to my friends and colleagues at the London College of Fashion for their encouragement and support during the preparation of this book. In particular, thanks are due to Karen Denison for organising salon time for the photo shoot.

I would like to thank my family for all their help and support; special thanks to Susie Robertson for her efforts in typing and preparing the manuscript, and for delivering it on time in spite of adverse circumstances.

Finally my grateful thanks to the following students for their time and patience while modelling for the photographs:
Emma Avis, Lisa Barham, Nicola Christodulou and Georgina Vassili.

The publishers would like to thank the following for permission to reproduce copyright material: figure 1.1, Ronald Sheridan/Ancient Art & Architecture Collection; figure 1.2, British Library, London. The commissioned photographs were taken by Susan Ford.

British Library Cataloguing in Publication Data

Rosser, Mo
   Body massage : therapy basics
   1.Massage 2.Physical therapy
   I.Title
   615.8'22

   ISBN 0340658266

First published 1996
Impression number   10 9 8 7 6 5 4 3 2 1
Year   2000 1999 1998 1997 1996

Typeset by Wearset, Boldon, Tyne and Wear.
Printed in Great Britain for Hodder & Stoughton Educational, a division of Hodder Headline Plc, 338 Euston Road, London NW1 3BH by the Bath Press, Bath

Contents

· ·

Introduction

· ·

Massage is the manipulation of body tissues to produce therapeutic effects. Massage may be performed manually with the hands or mechanically using vibrating equipment. Manual massage is more personal and usually preferred by the clients, but mechanical techniques are useful when greater depth and vigour are required.

This text book provides the information, underpinning knowledge and practical guidelines which will ensure that all those interested in the study of massage will be equipped to practise in a hygienic, safe, effective and professional manner.

Massage has regained popularity over the past ten years as its many benefits have again been recognised and acknowledged. The general public is now very aware of the value of massage in combating the stresses and tensions of modern living. Athletes, sportspeople and dancers include massage in their training schedules to aid recovery and to prevent or treat soft tissue injuries. There are numerous opportunities and openings for the professional massage practitioner. Helping others, reducing stress, relieving pain and contributing to general health brings great personal satisfaction and a rewarding, fulfilling career.

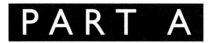

PART A

Underpinning knowledge

CHAPTER 1 Brief history of massage

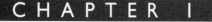

OBJECTIVES

After you have studied this chapter you will be able to:

1 explain how massage was used in ancient civilisations
2 explain the derivation of the word 'massage'
3 describe the development of massage from ancient to modern times
4 explain why massage became little used as a therapeutic treatment in hospitals
5 discuss the development of massage in the beauty and leisure industries.

Massage has been practised throughout the centuries since the earliest civilisations. It has been used medically as a therapeutic healing treatment and also for invigorating, soothing and beautifying the body. Massage or rubbing is an instinctive act for relieving pain and discomfort, and for soothing and calming. The use of fats and aromatic oils for anointing and lubricating the body are referred to in the Bible and the Koran.

The word 'massage' has its origin in the Arabian word *mass* or *mass'h*, which means 'to press gently'. The Greek word *massage* means 'to knead' and the French word *masser* means 'to massage'.

Massage in ancient times

The earliest evidence of massage being used is found in the cave paintings of ancient cave dwellers. These wall drawings and paintings show people massaging each other. Various artefacts also found contain traces of fats and oils mixed with herbs. These indicate that lubricants may have been used, perhaps for healing, soothing or beautifying purposes.

As early as 3000 BC, the Chinese practised massage to cure ailments and improve general health. Records of this can be found in the British Museum. Ancient Chinese books record lists of massage movements with descriptions of their technique. One of these books, *The Cong Fau of Tao-Tse*, also contains lists of exercises and massage used to improve general health and well-being. The Chinese found that pressure techniques were very effective on specific points and they developed special techniques called *amma* (see figure 1.1). This was the beginning of the development of acupressure and acupuncture.

These massage techniques spread to Japan where they were further developed. The Japanese used similar pressure techniques on specific points which they called *tsubo*. This form of massage has been practised over the centuries; it has recently regained recognition and popularity and is now known as *Shiatsu*. Many therapists have studied these techniques, which they combine with other forms of treatment for the benefit of their clients.

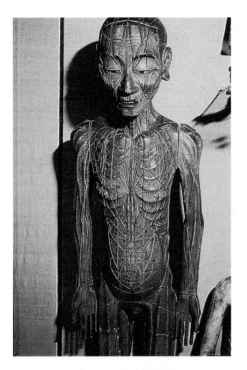

Figure 1.1 An ancient Chinese acupuncture and massage study figure, showing treatments points.

Records show that the Hindus practised massage as part of their hygiene routines. A sacred book called the *Ayur-Veda* (The Art of Life), which was written around 1800 BC, describes how shampooing and rubbing were used to reduce fatigue and promote well-being and cleanliness.

The Egyptians and Persians used massage for cosmetic as well as therapeutic effects (see figure 1.2). They mixed fats, oils, herbs and resins for care of the skin and beautifying the body and face. Pots and jars containing these creams have been found in Egyptian tombs. Cleopatra is said to have bathed in milk and then to have been massaged with aromatic oils and creams by her handmaidens.

The practice of massage spread from the East into Europe, where it was well established by 500 BC.

Massage in Classical Greece and Rome

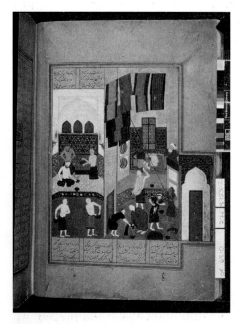

Figure 1.2 This ancient Persian document shows bathing and massage in a Turkish bath

The Greeks believed in the cultivation of a healthy mind and body, which is similar to the 'holistic approach' practised by many people today. Rituals of bathing, massage, exercise or dancing were practised by men and women. They encouraged the pursuit of physical fitness and organised regular sporting, gymnastic and athletic competitions. Massage was used before events to improve performance and after events to relieve fatigue and aid recovery. Gladiators and soldiers were massaged before battle to give vigour and promote fitness and health, and afterwards to aid recovery, healing and relaxation. Homer writes in the poem *The Odyssey* of Greek soldiers being rubbed with oils and anointed by beautiful women to aid their recovery and regain strength on return from battle.

Around 500 BC the Greek physician Herodicus used massage with oils and herbs to treat medical conditions and diseases. Hippocrates, who is now thought of as the father of medicine, was a pupil of Herodicus. He began to study the effects of massage on his patients. He concluded and recorded that 'hard rubbing binds, soft rubbing loosens, much rubbing causes parts to waste but moderate rubbing makes them grow'. Hippocrates also concluded that it was more beneficial to apply pressure in an upward direction, i.e. towards the heart, as we practise today. In Hippocrates's day, the function of the heart and the circulation of the blood was not known. It is therefore remarkable that he reached this conclusion only by observing the effect on the tissues of different strokes. With our knowledge of the heart and circulating blood we understand why pressure upwards is more beneficial: the condition of the tissues improves because deoxygenated blood and waste products are removed quickly as massage speeds up blood and lymph flow. Even without the benefit of this knowledge, Hippocrates taught his pupils that massage movements should be performed with pressure upwards to promote healing.

The Romans followed similar routines to the Greeks. They practised bathing, exercise and massage for health and social relaxation. Large private and public baths were built. These included water baths and steam rooms, gymnasium and massage areas. The baths were maintained at different temperatures and progress was made from cold to hot baths. Wealthy Romans would use these daily for cleansing, exercising, relaxing and socialising. Servants were always in attendance, with oils and creams to massage their masters when required. The Romans built similar baths in the countries that were conquered by their armies. Many such baths were built after the Roman conquest of Britain in 55 BC, and their ruins can be seen in Britain today in towns and cities such as Bath, Caerleon and St Albans. Massage techniques recorded from those times include manipulations known as squeezing, pinching or pummelling. They relate to the petrissage and percussion movements used today.

The Dark Ages to the Renaissance

Little is known about massage or health and beauty practices throughout the Dark and Middle Ages, i.e. from the decline of the Roman Empire around 500 AD until the Middle Ages around 1400 AD. Few records remain from those days of wars, strict religions, superstition and persecution. Little value was placed on education, the arts, physical health and fitness.

Following this period came the Renaissance (rebirth) in 1450 AD. Interest in the arts and sciences flourished and there was renewed interest in health practices. Once again we see massage advocated and practised for therapeutic purposes.

In the sixteenth century, the French surgeon Ambroise Paré (1517–90) promoted and developed the use of massage. He was the personal physician to four French kings. He is reputed to have successfully treated Mary Queen of Scots with massage. Paré graded massage into gentle, medium and vigorous. We use similar categories today, namely soothing or relaxing, general, and stimulating. Many other physicians copied his methods and massage was established medically.

The development of modern massage techniques

Modern massage techniques have evolved mainly from a system developed by a Swedish physiologist called Per Henrik Ling (1776–1839). He developed a system of passive and active exercises known as 'Swedish Remedial Gymnastics' and also a system of massage movements. Ling used the terms 'effleurage', 'petrissage', 'vibration', 'friction', 'rolling' and 'slapping'. Most of these terms are still used today, but some changes and modifications have been made in the groupings and names of manipulations.

Dr Johann Mezgner (1839–1909), a Dutch physician, developed massage for use in rehabilitation and used it to successfully treat many diseases and disorders. He adapted massage techniques in the light of his knowledge of anatomy and physiology. His theories, based on sound scientific principles, became accepted as medical practice and gained him many followers, particularly in Germany and America.

The work of Ling and Mezgner established massage as an effective therapeutic treatment. Techniques were taught in medical schools and the beneficial effects became widely recognised and accepted in the medical field. In England, the eminent surgeon John Grosvenor (1742–1823) used massage to treat joints. He recommended massage for the treatment of rheumatism, gout and stiffness of joints.

Nurses were encouraged to train and use massage for the treatment of patients, under the guidance of doctors. In 1894 a group of women founded the 'Society of Trained Masseuses'. Rules and regulations for training and examinations for qualifying were established. These women raised standards and fought to establish massage therapy as a reputable profession.

Twentieth-century developments

During the First World War the demand for massage to treat the injured grew and many more massage therapists were trained. Membership of the Society of Trained Masseuses grew and in 1920 it amalgamated with the 'Institute of Massage and Remedial Exercise'. In recognition of the valuable work contributed by its members during the war, a Royal Charter was granted and the title was changed to the 'Chartered Society of Massage and Medical Gymnastics'. The title was changed again in 1943 and became the 'Chartered Society of Physiotherapy'. In 1964 its members became State Registered. This protected and gave status to those qualified therapists who were practising in clinics and hospitals, and made it impossible for those without a recognised qualification to practise.

With the development of alternative electrical-based treatments, the use of massage to treat medical conditions declined. There was rapid growth in electrotherapy and eventually massage ceased to be part of physiotherapy training. It became little used as a therapeutic treatment in hospitals. There was, however, a continuing demand for massage in clinics, health farms, fitness and leisure centres.

In 1966 the City and Guilds of London Institute explored the possibility of establishing a course in beauty therapy to include massage. This course would provide thorough training, background knowledge and a recognised professional qualification which ensured a high standard of practice. In 1968 the first full-time course was offered in colleges of further education. The British Association of Beauty Therapists and Cosmetologists, the International Health and Beauty Council and other organisations also developed courses and offered certificates and diplomas. The growth in complementary medicine and the holistic approach to health has increased the demands for well-qualified practitioners, not only in massage but also in aromatherapy, reflexology, shiatsu, etc. Courses are now validated by the Health and Beauty Therapy Training

Board and therapists must meet the criteria of the National Council of Vocational Qualifications.

?

1 Outline the evidence which indicates that massage was practised by cave dwellers.

2 Name three languages from which the word 'massage' may have derived.

3 Explain briefly what is meant by the Chinese technique of acupuncture.

4 Describe briefly how the Greeks and Romans incorporated massage into their rituals.

5 Name the Greek physician who concluded that massage pressure should be applied in an upward direction.

6 Exlain why little is known about massage in the Dark Ages.

7 Name three eminent doctors who promoted massage for healing purposes.

8 Explain why the reputation of massage grew during and after the First World War.

9 Name the examining body that established the first beauty therapy course in colleges of further and higher education.

CHAPTER 2

Body systems and the physiological and psychological effects of massage

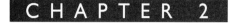

OBJECTIVES

After you have studied this chapter you will be able to:

1 describe the organisational levels of the body
2 list the classification of tissues
3 list the types of epithelial tissue and state where they are found
4 list the types of connective tissue and give their function
5 list the body systems and
   (a) describe the main body systems relevant to massage
   (b) explain the functions of these systems
   (c) explain the physiological effects of massage on the main body systems
   (d) explain the psychological effects of massage.

Physiological effects are the effects on the structure and function of the body. Psychological effects are the effects on the mental state.

Before describing these effects it is necessary to have a basic understanding of the structure and function of body systems. This underpinning knowledge will enable the therapist to understand and explain the effects of massage. Unfortunately an in-depth study of anatomy and physiology is not within the scope of this book. The following are brief summaries of the relevant systems. (The anatomy of specific body parts is discussed in Chapter 8.)

Organisational levels

The organisational levels of the body are chemical, cell, tissue, organ and system.

◆ At the very basic level are the **chemicals** which are essential for maintaining life. These chemicals combine to form cells.

◆ The **cells** are the basic structural and functional units of the body. All the activities which maintain life are carried out by the cells. The body is made up of billions of cells; they all have a similar structure but are modified to suit their function.

◆ Groups of similar cells form the **tissues** of the body, e.g. epithelial tissue covers and lines structures.

◆ Different tissues group together to form the **organs** of the body. Each organ will perform a specific function, e.g. the heart pumps blood around the body.

◆ Many different organs link together to form the **systems** of the body. They work together to carry out an essential function, e.g. the digestive system deals with food.

CELLS

The parts common to all cells are:

1 **plasma membrane**: outer layer protects, gives shape and separates the material inside the cell from that outside; it regulates the movement of substances in and out of the cells

2 **cytoplasm**: jelly-like substance within the membrane

3 **organelles**: mini organs in the cytoplasm that carry out the functions of the cell; the main one is the nucleus, known as the control centre

4 **inclusions**: chemical substances in the cytoplasm, e.g. melanin and glycogen.

Characteristics of cells are metabolism, respiration, growth, reproduction, excretion, irritability and movement.

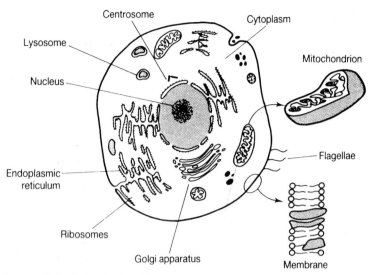

Figure 2.1 A typical cell

Tissues

Groups of similar cells are organised together to form the body tissues. The cells of one tissue will all be the same, but they will be different for the different tissues. Tissues are classified into four types: epithelial, connective, muscular and nervous.

Table 2.1 Classification of tissues

Epithelial	Simple	Squamous – flat cells – lines heart, blood vessels, etc.
		Cuboidal – cube shaped – lines ducts of glands
		Columnar – column shaped – lines stomach and body tracts
		Columnar ciliated – columns with hairs – lines respiratory tract
	Compound	Squamous – layers of flat cells – lines mouth
		Cuboidal – ducts of sweat glands
		Columnar – lines male urethra and anus
		Transitional – lines bladder
	Glandular	Secreting cells found in glands
Connective tissue	Areolar	Connecting skin to tissues and muscles
	Adipose	Stores fat under skin and around organs
	Dense fibrous	Gives tensile strength – ligaments and tendons
	Yellow elastic	Gives elasticity to skin and walls of arteries
	Reticular	Found in lymphatic tissue
	Cartilage	Fibro-cartilage – intervertebral discs
		Elastic cartilage – outer ear
		Hyaline cartilage – covers the ends of bones at joints

Table 2.1 continued

	Bone	Compact – outer layer of bones
		Cancellous – inner mass of bones
	Blood	Fluid connective tissue; transports substances around body and regulates body temperature
Muscular tissue	Skeletal	Produces body movement, maintains posture and produces heat
	Cardiac	Heart muscle maintains pumping action
	Smooth	Walls of blood vessels and intestines – peristalsis
Nervous tissue	Neurones	Pick up stimuli and conduct impulses to other neurones, muscle fibres or glands
	Neuroglia	Supporting substance which protects neurones
Membranes (four types)	Cutaneous	Skin
	Mucous	Lines body tracts which open to exterior – respiratory and gastro-intestinal
	Serous	Lines body cavities, thorax and surrounds lungs
	Synovial	Lines joints but not the cartilage

BODY ORGANS

Many tissues will be organised to form the organs of the body. Each organ has a specific function or functions to perform, e.g. the stomach digests food, the lungs exchange gases, the heart pumps blood, the kidneys form urine and filter fluids, and the ovaries produce and release ova. Organs form parts of the systems of the body.

BODY SYSTEMS

Each body system consists of many organs which link together to perform a common function. All the systems are interrelated and function together to maintain life. There are 11 body systems:

- integumentary
- skeletal
- muscular
- nervous
- cardio-vascular
- lymphatic
- respiratory
- digestive
- urinary
- reproductive
- endocrine

Table 2.2 Classification of body systems

System	Structure	Function
Integumentary	The skin and all its structures – nails, hair, sweat and oil glands	Protects, regulates temperature, eliminates waste, makes vitamin D, receives stimuli
Skeletal	The bones, joints and cartilages	Supports, protects, aids movement, stores minerals, protects cells that produce blood cells
Muscular	Usually refers to skeletal muscle but includes cardiac and smooth	Produces movement, maintains posture and produces heat
Nervous	Brain, spinal cord, nerves and sense organs	Communicates and co-ordinates body functions
Cardio-vascular	Heart, blood vessels and blood	Transports substances around body, helps regulate body temperature and prevents blood loss by blood clotting
Lymphatic	Lymphatic vessels, nodes, lymph, spleen, tonsils and thymus gland	Returns proteins and plasma to blood. Carries fat from intestine to blood. Filters body fluid, forms white blood cells and protects against disease
Respiratory	Pharynx, larynx, trachea, bronchi and lungs	Supplies oxygen and removes carbon dioxide
Digestive	Gastro-intestinal tract, salivary glands, gall-bladder, liver and pancreas	Physical and chemical breakdown of food. Absorption of nutrients and elimination of waste
Urinary	Kidneys, ureters, bladder and urethra	Regulates chemical composition of blood. Helps to balance the acid/alkali content in the body and eliminates urine
Reproductive	All organs of reproduction – ovaries, testes, etc.	Involved in reproduction and production of sex hormones
Endocrine	All the hormone-producing ductless glands	Hormones regulate a wide variety of body activities, e.g. growth, and maintain body balance

Skeleton

The human skeleton is made up of 206 bones. These are grouped into two main divisions: the **axial skeleton** which forms the core or axis of the body, and the **appendicular skeleton** which forms the girdles and limbs. It is important to identify skeletal bones, particularly those with bony points or prominences which must be avoided when massaging.

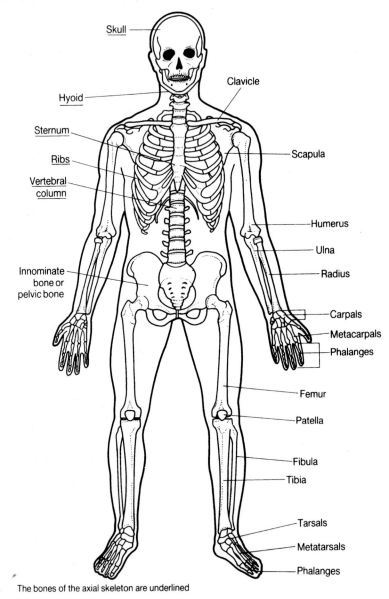

Skull

Clavicle

Hyoid

Sternum

Ribs

Vertebral column

Scapula

Humerus

Ulna

Radius

Innominate bone or pelvic bone

Carpals

Metacarpals

Phalanges

Femur

Patella

Fibula

Tibia

Tarsals

Metatarsals

Phalanges

The bones of the axial skeleton are underlined

Figure 2.2 The human skeleton

AXIAL SKELETON

The bones of the axial skeleton include the:

◆ skull (head)

◆ vertebral column (spine)

- sternum (breast bone)

- ribs

- hyoid bone (small bone in neck below mandible).

APPENDICULAR SKELETON

The bones of the appendicular skeleton include:

Upper limb
- clavicle (collar bone)

- scapula (shoulder bone)

- humerus (upper arm bone)

- radius (forearm – lateral)

- ulna (forearm – medial)

- carpals (wrist)

- metacarpals (palm)

- phalanges (fingers)

Lower limb
- innominate or pelvic bone (hip bone)

- femur (thigh bone)

- patella (knee cap)

- tibia (large bone of lower leg – medial)

- fibula (thin bone of lower leg – lateral)

- tarsals (ankle)

- metatarsals (foot)

- phalanges (toes).

VERTEBRAL COLUMN

The vertebral column (also known as the spinal column) is composed of 33 vertebrae. Some are fused together, making 26 bones. The vertebrae are separated by intervertebral discs of fibro-cartilage which act as shock absorbers. The bones and discs are bound together by strong ligaments.

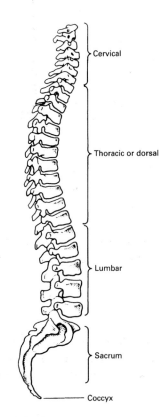

Figure 2.3 **The vertebral column**

The column is divided into five regions:

- ◆ **cervical**   7 vertebrae (neck), concave when viewed posteriorly

- ◆ **thoracic**   12 vertebrae (upper back), convex when viewed posteriorly

- ◆ **lumbar**   5 vertebrae (lower, small of back), concave when viewed posteriorly

- ◆ **sacral**   5 fused vertebrae (sacrum), convex when viewed posteriorly

- ◆ **coccygeal**   4 fused vertebrae (coccyx).

JOINTS

A joint is where two or more bones join or articulate. There are three main groups: fibrous, cartilaginous and synovial.

1 **Fibrous**: immovable joints; the bones fit tightly together and are held firmly by fibrous tissue. There is no joint cavity. Examples are the sutures of the skull.

2 **Cartilaginous**: slightly moveable joints; the bones are connected by a disc or plate of fibro-cartilage. There is no joint cavity. Examples are the symphysis pubis (between the pubic bones) and the intervertebral joints (between the vertebral bodies).

3 **Synovial**: freely moveable joints; these are the most numerous in the body. There are six different types of synovial joints. They are classified according to their planes of movement, which depends on the shape of the articulating bones. All the freely moveable joints of the body are synovial joints and, although their shape and movements vary, they all have certain characteristics in common:

(a) a **joint cavity** (space within the joint)

(b) a **synovial membrane** lining the capsule which produces synovial fluid

(c) **synovial fluid** or synovium – a viscous fluid which lubricates and nourishes the joint

(d) **hyaline cartilage** which covers the surfaces of the articulating bones. It is sometimes called articular cartilage. It reduces friction and allows smooth movement

(e) a **capsule**, or articulating capsule, which surrounds the joints like a sleeve. It holds the bones together and encloses the cavity. The capsule is strengthened on the outside by ligaments which help to stabilise and strengthen the joints. Ligaments may also be found inside a joint, holding bones together and increasing stability. Massage is used around joints to increase the circulation and to free ligaments which may have become bound down following injury.

DISCS (MENISCI)

Some joints have pads of fibro-cartilage called discs. They are attached to the bones and give the joint a better 'fit'. They also cushion movement, e.g. cartilages of the knee.

BURSAE

Any movement produces friction between the moving parts. In order to reduce friction, sac-like structures containing synovial fluid are found between tissues. These are called bursae and are usually found between tendons and bone.

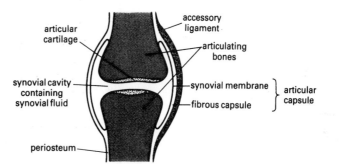

Figure 2.4 A synovial joint

CLASSIFICATION OF THE SIX SYNOVIAL JOINTS

1 **gliding joint**, e.g. intercarpal or intertarsal joints

2 **hinge joint**, e.g. elbow or knee

3 **pivot joint**, e.g. superior radio-ulnar joint or atlas on axis

4 **ellipsoid joint** (Condyloid), e.g. wrist or knuckle joints

5 **saddle joint**, e.g. base of the thumb

6 **ball-and-socket joint**, shoulder or hip joint

EFFECTS OF MASSAGE ON BONE TISSUE AND JOINTS

◆ Bones are covered by a layer of connective tissue known as the 'periosteum'. Blood vessels from the periosteum penetrate the bone. Deep massage movements will stimulate blood flow to the periosteum and hence increase blood supply to the bone.

◆ Massage around joints will increase the circulation and nourish the structures surrounding the joint.

◆ Massage is effective in loosening adhesions in structures around joints. For example, frictions across a ligament help to loosen it from underlying structures.

Muscle

Muscles form the body flesh. Their function is to produce movement, maintain posture and produce body heat. Muscle tissue is totally under the control of the nervous system; impulses transmitted from the brain via motor nerves initiate contraction of muscle fibres. This contraction pulls on bones and movement occurs at joints.

STRUCTURE OF SKELETAL MUSCLE

Skeletal muscle is composed of muscle fibres arranged in buntlles called **fasciculi**. Many bundles of fibres make up the complete muscle. The fibres, bundles and muscles are surrounded and protected by connective tissue sheaths.

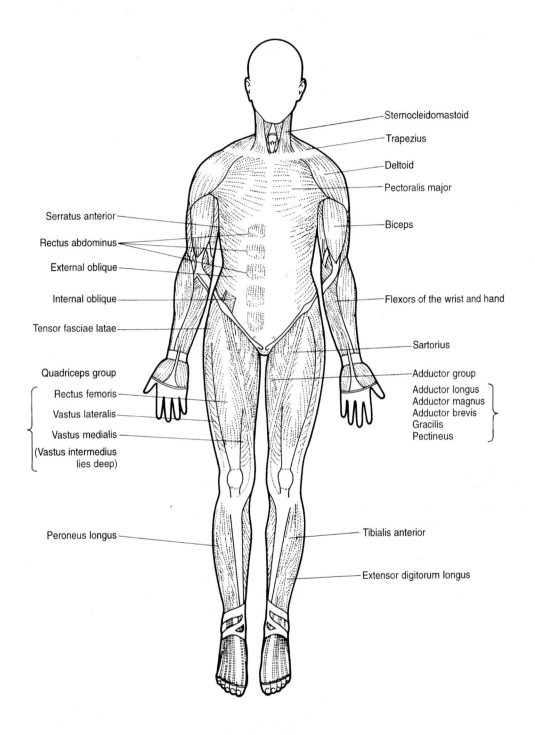

Figure 2.5a Muscles of the body – anterior

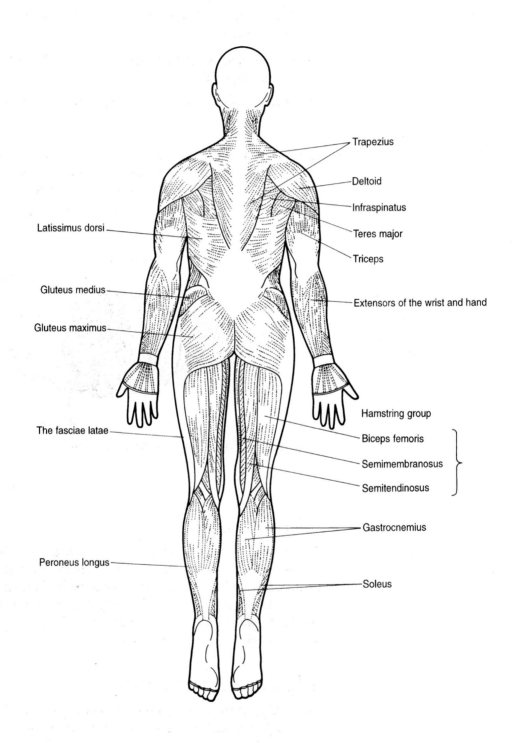

Trapezius

Deltoid

Infraspinatus

Teres major

Triceps

Latissimus dorsi

Extensors of the wrist and hand

Gluteus medius

Gluteus maximus

Hamstring group

Biceps femoris

Semimembranosus

Semitendinosus

The fasciae latae

Gastrocnemius

Peroneus longus

Soleus

Figure 2.5b Muscles of the body – posterior

♦ The connective tissue around each fibre is called the **endomysium**.

♦ The connective tissue around each bundle is called the **perimysium**.

♦ The connective tissue around the muscle is called the **epimysium**.

If this connective tissue becomes tight or adheres to underlying structures, the petrissage movements are very effective in freeing and stretching the tissue, allowing the muscle fibres to function normally.

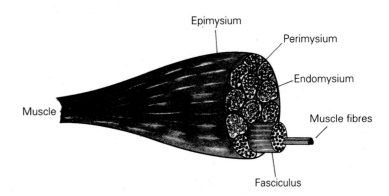

Epimysium

Perimysium

Endomysium

Muscle

Muscle fibres

Fasciculus

Figure 2.6 The structure of skeletal muscle

Muscle fibres

Muscle fibres are long, thin, multi-nucleated cells. The fibres vary from 10 to 100 microns in diameter, and from a few millimetres to many centimetres in length. The long fibres extend the full length of the muscle while the short fibres end in connective tissue intersections within the muscle.

Muscle attachments

As previously explained, a muscle is composed of muscle fibres and connective tissue components – the endomysium, perimysium and epimysium. Certain muscles have connective tissue intersections dividing the muscle into several bellies, as seen in *rectus abdominis.*

These sheets of connective tissue blend at either end of the muscle and attach the muscle to underlying bones. Muscles are attached via tendons or aponeuroses.

◆ **Tendons** are tough cord-like structures of connective tissue which attach muscles to bones.

◆ **Aponeuroses** are flat sheets of connective tissue which attach muscles along the length of bone.

A muscle has at least two points of attachment known as the origin and insertion of the muscle.

◆ The **origin** is usually proximal and stationary or immovable.

◆ The **insertion** is usually distal and moveable.

Following over-use or injury, these tendons may become inflamed. Massage around the area can restore function. Transverse frictions are useful for freeing tendons held by adhesions.

MUSCLE SHAPE

Muscle shape varies depending on the function of the muscle. The fleshy bulk of the muscle is known as the belly. The muscle fibres forming bundles lie parallel or obliquely to the line of pull of the muscle. Parallel fibres

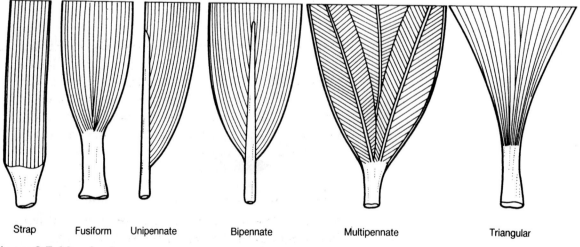

| Strap | Fusiform | Unipennate | Bipennate | Multipennate | Triangular |

Figure 2.7 Muscle shapes

are found in strap-like and fusiform muscles. These long fibres allow for a wide range of movement. Oblique fibres are found in triangular and pennate muscles. These shorter fibres are found where muscle strength is required.

BLOOD SUPPLY TO SKELETAL MUSCLE

Supplies of oxygen and nutrients required by muscles are brought by the blood via the arteries supplying the muscle; the waste products are removed via the veins. The arteries branch to form smaller arteries and arterioles within the perimysium. They then further divide forming capillary networks within the endomysium, where they join venules which lead to veins. When muscles are relaxed, the capillary network delivers blood to the muscle fibres. When muscles contract, the pressure impedes the flow of blood through the capillary beds, which reduces the supply of oxygen and nutrients and limits removal of waste. During exercise, muscle fibres alternately contract and relax, and the capillaries deliver blood during the relaxation phase. However, repeated or sustained contractions, such as isometric work or exercising without sufficient rest periods, prevent blood flow to the muscle fibres due to compression on blood vessels and capillaries. This results in **muscle fatigue**, due to lack of oxygen and nutrients and the accumulation of waste products such as lactic acid. The strength and speed of contraction becomes progressively weaker until the muscle finally fails to relax completely, resulting in muscle spasm and pain.

Long effleurage strokes speed up venous return and the circulation to the muscle is increased. Accumulated waste is removed and pain and stiffness relieved. The squeezing movements of petrissage also increase the circulation. When tension in the muscle is relieved, pressure is decreased and circulation flows normally through the capillary beds.

MUSCLE TONE

Muscle tone is the state of partial contraction or tension found in muscles even when at rest. Only a small number of muscle fibres will be in a state of contraction.

This is sufficient to produce tautness in the muscle but not to result in full contraction and movement. Different groups of fibres contract alternately, working a 'shift' system to prevent fatigue. Changes in muscle tone are adjusted according to the information received from sensory receptors within the muscles and their tendons. **Muscle spindles** transmit information on the degree of stretch within the muscle. **Tendon receptors** called golgi organs transmit information on the amount of tension applied to the tendon by muscle contraction. Too much stretch and tension will result in reduction in muscle tone. Too little will result in increase in muscle tone. Muscle tone is essential for maintaining upright postures.

◆ Hypotonic muscles, i.e. those with less than the normal degree of tone, are said to be **flaccid**.

◆ Hypertonic muscles, i.e. those with greater than normal degree of tone, are said to be **spastic**.

Massage aids the relaxation of muscles due to the warmth created, reflex response and removal of accumulated waste.

EFFECTS OF MASSAGE ON MUSCLE TISSUE

◆ The blood supply to muscles is increased. Deoxygenated blood and waste is removed and fresh oxygenated blood and nutrients are brought to the muscles. The metabolic rate is increased and the condition of the muscles will improve.

◆ Massage will reduce pain, stiffness and muscle fatigue produced by the accumulation of waste following anaerobic contraction. The removal of this metabolic waste, i.e. lactic acid and carbon dioxide, is speeded up and normal function is more quickly restored. This is particularly important following hard training, sport and athletic performance, for example, when massage will speed up the recovery of muscles, allowing the athlete to return to training more quickly. The increased nutrients and oxygen will also facilitate tissue repair and recovery.

◆ Massage warms muscles due to the increased blood flow, the friction of the hands moving over the area and the friction of the tissues as they move over each other. This reduces tension and aids relaxation of the muscles. Warm muscles contract more efficiently and are more extensile than cold muscles. Thus performance is enhanced and the likelihood of strains, sprains, micro-tears or other injury is reduced. Massage prior to exercise must be used in conjunction with (but not instead of) warm-up and stretch exercise.

◆ The elasticity of muscles is improved because manipulations such as kneading, wringing and picking up stretch the fibres and separate the bundles. Any restricting fibrous adhesions are broken down and any tight fascia surrounding the bundles are stretched, allowing muscle fibres to function normally.

◆ Massage will break down adhesions and fibrositic nodules which may have developed within the muscle as a result of tension, poor posture or injury.

Skin

The skin forms a protective covering over the entire surface of the body; it is continuous with the membranes lining the orifices. It covers a surface area of approximately two square metres, and varies in thickness from 0.05 mm to 3 mm, being thickest on the soles of the feet and palms of the hands and thinnest on the lips, eyelids, inner surfaces of the limbs and on the abdomen. The skin includes hair, nails, glands and various sensory receptors.

SKIN COLOUR

Skin colour varies from person to person and from race to race. Skin colour is due to the pigment melanin, to the quantity of blood flowing through the blood vessels, and to the pigment carotene which is present in the skin of certain races such as Asians. The number of melanocytes is approximately the same in all races, but colour varies because of the amount and type of melanin produced.

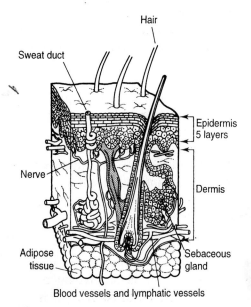

Hair

Sweat duct

Epidermis
5 layers

Nerve

Dermis

Adipose
tissue

Sebaceous
gland

Blood vessels and lymphatic vessels

**Figure 2.8 Cross-section through
the skin**

SKIN STRUCTURE

The skin is composed of two main layers with a
subcutaneous fatty layer underneath. The two main
layers are:

◆ epidermis

◆ dermis.

These layers may be further subdivided as follows.

1 The epidermis has five layers:

   (a) stratum corneum (superficial layer)

   (b) stratum lucidum

   (c) stratum granulosum

   (d) stratum spinosum

   (e) stratum basale (germinativum) (deepest layer).

2 The dermis has two layers:

   (a) papillary layer

   (b) reticular layer.

EPIDERMIS

The epidermis is composed of five layers of stratified
squamous epithelium. The living cells of the two
deepest layers contain nuclei; the dead cells of the
upper three layers lose their nuclei and become filled
with a protein called **keratin**. As the cells multiply they
push upward, forming the next layer.

STRATUM BASALE (STRATUM GERMINATIVUM)

This is the deepest layer of the epidermis. It is a single
layer of cells on a basement membrane and lies directly
on the papillary layer of the dermis. The capillary
network of the dermis provides nutrients for these living
cells. The cells have a nucleus and multiply by mitosis.
Approximately one in ten of these basal cells are
specialised cells called melanocytes. They produce the
pigment melanin from the amino acid tyrosine. Melanin
is produced to protect the cells against the damaging
effect of ultra-violet radiation. It gives the skin its brown

colour. This layer also contains the nerve endings sensitive to touch (Merkel's discs).

STRATUM SPINOSUM

This is composed of eight to ten layers of living cells. Granules of melanin pass into this layer. The cells begin to lose their shape and have projections or spines which join the cells together.

STRATUM GRANULOSUM

This consists of three to five layers of flattened cells. Enzymes break down the nucleus and the cells die. Keratohyaline is laid down in the cytoplasm, giving the first stages of keratinisation. The protein keratin protects the skin from injury and invasion of micro-organisms and makes it waterproof.

STRATUM LUCIDUM

This is composed of several layers of clear, flat, dead cells that are translucent and filled with keratin. This layer is found only on the palms of the hands and soles of the feet.

STRATUM CORNEUM

This is the superficial layer, composed of many rows of flat, dead, scaly cells filled with keratin that are constantly shed and replaced (this shedding of cells is known as desquamation). Sebum secreted by the sebaceous glands helps to keep this layer soft and supple.

DERMIS

The dermis lies under the epidermis and is composed of two layers: the upper papillary layer and the lower reticular layer.

The surface of the papillary layer is ridged, forming an uneven surface. These finger-like projections increase the surface area and are called **dermal papillae**. They produce the pattern known as finger prints. The blood capillary loops of the dermis transport nutrients and oxygen to basal layer cells and remove waste products.

Some elastin and collagen fibres are found in the matrix.

The reticular layer is composed of dense irregular connective tissue with more collagen and elastin fibres. This gives the skin strength, extensibility and elasticity. The skin's ability to stretch and recoil is necessary during pregnancy and obesity. The ground substance or matrix retains water, helping the skin to remain firm and turgid.

Many structures are found in the dermis. They include blood vessels, lymphatic vessels, sebaceous glands, sweat glands, nerves and nerve endings, hair in hair follicles, erector pili muscles, fibres (white fibres and yellow elastic fibres), fibroblasts, mast cells, plasma cells and macrophages.

BLOOD VESSELS

The dermis is well supplied with blood vessels, partly to provide nutrients to the actively dividing cells of the epidermis (which has no direct supply), but also to enable the skin to play its part in the regulation of body temperature. Small vessels leave the dermal plexus at right angles and pass upwards to the skin's surface, ending in the dermal papillae. Nutrients and oxygen pass out into the tissue fluid and into the basal cells, and waste products pass out of the cells into tissue fluid through capillaries to the small veins.

The amount of blood flowing near the surface of the skin is controlled by nerve endings in the artery walls. If the body is becoming too hot, the small arteries dilate (get bigger). This causes flushing of the skin or **erythema** and the body loses heat via the skin. If the body becomes too cool the arteries constrict, preventing heat loss. Massage stimulates the nerve endings and by reflex action the blood vessels dilate.

LYMPHATIC VESSELS

There is a network of fine lymphatic capillaries and vessels throughout the dermis. They are blind-end tubes with walls of greater permeability than blood capillaries – larger particles can enter these vessels and be drained away in the lymph. The broken down products of infection by micro-organisms are also drained away in the lymph.

SEBACEOUS GLANDS

These glands secrete an oily substance called **sebum**. (It consists mainly of waxes, fats and fatty acids, and dehydrocholesterol which forms vitamin D in sunlight.) The glands are found in all areas except the soles and palms and between the fingers and toes. They are numerous on the scalp, forehead, nose, chin, chest and between the shoulders. The glands are sac-like and are usually attached to the side wall of hair follicles into which the secretions enter via a duct, but some open directly onto the skin surface.

The glands are composed of epithelial cells which multiply, grow larger towards the centre and become filled with sebum. Eventually they burst, discharging sebum into the hair follicle. The production of sebum is controlled by hormones (secreted by the endocrine glands). Hormonal imbalance, for example at puberty, increases the flow of sebum, often causing problems such as acne.

The function of the sebum is to coat the skin and hair and keep the surface smooth and supple. It prevents loss of water from the skin. It also has antiseptic and anti-fungal properties, protecting the skin from bacterial and fungal infections. Sebum is gradually lost by washing and desquamation but is continually replaced. Massage stimulates the glands to produce more sebum.

Together with the sweat secreted by sweat glands, sebum forms a coating on the skin known as the **acid mantle** because the secretions have a pH of between 4.5 and 6 (acidic). This is neutralised when the skin is washed with soap (alkali), but is restored if all the soap is rinsed away.

SWEAT GLANDS

There are two types of sweat glands.

█ **Eccrine glands** (sudoriferous): these consist of a

coiled tube lying in the dermis with a straight duct opening in a pore on the skin surface. They are most numerous on the soles of feet and palms of hands. Sweat is a clear liquid containing 98% water, 2% sodium chloride and other substances, including urea and lactic acid. Sweat takes heat from the skin during evaporation. It therefore helps to maintain constant body temperature. Massage produces heat and therefore stimulates the sweat glands to produce more sweat.

2 **Apocrine glands** (odoriferous glands): these consist of coiled tubes larger than eccrine glands. They open into hair follicles, usually above the sebaceous glands. Sometimes they open directly onto the skin surface near a follicle. They are found in limited areas only, e.g. armpits and pubic areas. Development takes place at puberty. The secretion is somewhat viscous and sticky; when this is acted on by bacteria it leads to unpleasant body odour (BO).

NERVES

The nerves of the skin are mostly sensory. Most of the nerve endings lie in the dermis, but a few detecting pain lie in the lower layers of the epidermis. There are various types of nerve endings, modified according to their function. They detect cold, heat, pain and pressure (Meissner's corpuscles – touch; Pacinian corpuscles – deep pressure). The few motor nerves control secretion of sweat and contraction of erector pili muscles. These nerve endings may be soothed by massage, but if the massage is too light they may be irritated and if it is too deep, pain is increased. These factors will increase tension and must be avoided.

HAIR

Hairs are dead, horny structures composed of keratinised cells. They are found all over the body except on the soles and palms. They vary in length, texture and colour. Hairs are embedded in a depression called a hair follicle. The hair follicle consists of epithelial cells which form a tube passing obliquely into the dermis. It encases the hair bulb and hair root. The hair bulb is the expanded part of the hair which lies at the base of the follicle in the dermis. The hair root grows from the bulb and up through the follicle to the skin's surface. The hair shaft is the part which extends beyond the surface of the skin. Massage is more comfortable if it is performed in the direction of the hair growth, but this is not always possible.

ERECTOR PILI MUSCLES

These are small involuntary muscles connected to the hair follicles. When they contract they pull the hair follicles straight. This happens during extreme fright or cold – the skin around the follicle becomes raised, forming 'goose flesh'.

FIBRES

These consist of white collagen fibres and yellow elastic fibres.

White fibres are formed from non-elastic fibres of the protein collagen, lying in layers. They give the skin tensile strength and flexibility, and they bind structures together.

Yellow elastic fibres are formed from the protein elastin. They are scattered throughout the matrix. These highly elastic fibres are capable of stretch and recoil. They give the skin elasticity, enabling it to stretch and return to normal. This is important for pregnancy and obesity. If the skin is over-stretched small tears occur in the dermis. These can be seen as white lines called 'stretch marks'. All fibres are embedded in a jelly-like matrix. This is capable of absorbing water, giving firmness to the skin.

CELLS

1. Fibroblasts produce the matrix and fibres.

2. Mast cells release **histamine** following injury or reaction to an allergen. Histamine initiates an inflammatory response, causing dilation of capillaries and increasing the permeability of cell walls. This process aids tissue repair.

3. Plasma cells produce antibodies.

4 Leucocytes destroy and protect the body against micro-organisms.

5 Macrophages clean up cellular debris.

FUNCTIONS OF THE SKIN

◆ sensitivity (nerve endings and receptors)

◆ heat regulation (regulation of body temperature)

◆ absorption

◆ protection

◆ excretion

◆ secretion and storage

◆ vitamin D formation

EFFECTS OF MASSAGE ON THE SKIN

◆ Massage improves the condition of the skin because the increased blood supply increases the delivery of nutrients and oxygen and speeds up the removal of metabolic waste. Metabolism is increased which stimulates the cells of the stratum basale and increases mitosis (cell division). More cells move upwards towards the surface, improving the condition of the skin as old cells are replaced.

◆ Massage aids desquamation (shedding of dead cells). Increased mitosis will increase the shedding of the flaky dead cells of the stratum corneum. Also, the friction of the hands on the skin will rub off these dead cells on the surface.

◆ The colour of the skin is improved. Massage produces dilation of surface capillaries; this results in hyperaemia and erythema which improves the colour of sallow skin.

◆ Sebaceous glands are stimulated to produce and release more sebum. This lubricates the skin and keeps it soft and supple.

◆ The oil or cream used as a medium also lubricates and softens the skin.

◆ Sweat glands are stimulated to produce more sweat which aids cleansing and elimination of waste.

EFFECTS OF MASSAGE ON ADIPOSE TISSUE

Adipose tissue is composed of specialised cells called adipocytes, adapted to store fat. It is found under the skin in the subcutaneous layer and around organs. Fat is the body's energy reserve. It is stored when energy intake is greater than energy output and utilised if energy intake is less than energy output. Therefore, the only way of losing fat is through sensible eating and increasing activity or exercise. However, massage is thought to help the dispersal of fat because the deeper movements stimulate blood flow to the area. This softens the area and speeds up removal via the circulating blood.

The effects of massage on cellulite (very hard consolidated fat) is dealt with in Chapter 9.

Cardio-vascular system

The cardio-vascular (blood circulatory) system is a closed circuit. It is composed of a pump called the heart, a network of interconnecting tubes called blood

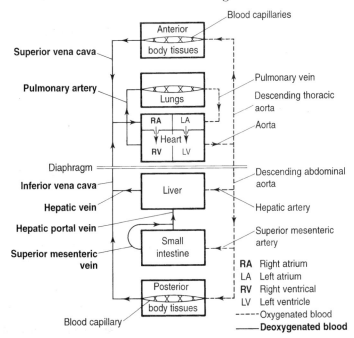

Figure 2.9 Circulation of blood

vessels, and the fluid flowing through the circuit known as blood. The parts which make up the system are:

◆ heart

◆ arteries and arterioles

◆ veins and venules

◆ capillaries

◆ blood.

The system is designed to carry blood to and from the organs and cells of the body. Blood carries oxygen, nutrients, hormones and enzymes to the cells, and takes away the waste products of metabolism from the cells.

TISSUE FLUID

All body cells are bathed in interstitial fluid (tissue fluid). This fluid provides a medium for substances to move across from the blood to the cells and from the cells to the blood. Oxygenated blood flows from the heart, through the arteries and arterioles, and into the capillaries. The walls of the capillaries are very thin; consequently the oxygen and nutrients pass out through the walls into the tissue fluid and from there into the cells. The waste products of metabolism pass out of the cells into the tissue fluid and into the capillaries in the same way. This deoxygenated blood is transported via the venules and veins back to the heart. The heart then pumps it to the lungs to be reoxygenated.

HEART

The heart lies in the thoracic cavity between the lungs. It is somewhat cone shaped, with the base above and the apex below. The walls of the heart are made up of three layers:

◆ **pericardium**: a tough outer coat of fibrous tissue

◆ **myocardium**: the middle coat of cardiac muscle

◆ **endocardium**: the inner lining of squamous epithelium.

The heart is divided into a right and left side by a muscular wall or septum. The left side of the heart deals with **oxygenated** blood. The right side deals with **deoxygenated** blood. Each side is further divided into two chambers separated by valves. The upper chambers are called **atria** (singular: atrium), the lower chambers are called **ventricles**.

FLOW OF BLOOD THROUGH THE HEART

◆ The inferior and superior venae cavae (veins) collect deoxygenated blood from the body and empty it into the right atrium.

◆ This blood then passes through the tricuspid valve into the right ventricle.

◆ From the right ventricle it is pumped into the pulmonary artery (the only artery carrying deoxygenated blood) and carried to the lungs.

◆ Interchange of gases occurs in the lungs and the oxygenated blood is carried by the pulmonary vein (the only vein carrying oxygenated blood) back to the left atrium of the heart.

◆ This blood passes through the bicuspid valve into the left ventricle.

◆ From the left ventricle blood is pumped into the aorta – the first artery of the general circulation. The aorta branches into numerous arteries which carry oxygenated blood to all body parts.

BLOOD VESSELS

There are three main types of blood vessels: arteries, veins and capillaries.

Arteries transport blood away from the heart to body tissues and organs. They carry nutrients and oxygenated blood (except the pulmonary artery which carries deoxygenated blood from the heart to the lungs). Artery walls are made up of three layers of tissues: a fibrous outer coat; a muscular middle coat and an inner lining of epithelium. These surround a centre core called the lumen. The lumen of arteries is smaller than that of veins and the middle muscular layer is thicker.

The aorta and arteries near the heart are large, but these branch many times and become smaller until they end as very small arterioles with thin walls. Blood is pumped through the arteries by the contraction of the heart.

Veins transport deoxygenated blood back to the heart. The walls are similar in structure to those of arteries but the middle muscular layer is thinner. The inner layer of epithelial cells is folded to form valves. These valves prevent the backward flow of blood. The lumen of veins is larger than that of arteries.

Blood is pumped along the veins by the contraction and relaxation of muscles and by the expansion and contraction of the thorax and diaphragm during breathing. If muscles are not contracting, e.g. during long periods of standing and inactivity, gravity exerts a downward force. If the valves are weak, blood 'pools' in the veins. This pressure overloads the veins and the wall bulges outwards, causing the condition known as varicose veins. Regular leg massage speeds up the flow of blood through the veins. This prevents overloading of the veins which helps prevent varicose veins.

Capillaries are thin-walled, tiny vessels which form networks among the tissue spaces. Arterioles enter capillary networks and venules leave. The primary function of capillaries is to allow the exchange of gases, nutrients and metabolic waste between the cells and the blood. Arterioles bring oxygen and nutrients to the capillaries. These pass through the thin vessel walls into the tissue fluid and then through the cell wall into the cell. Carbon dioxide and metabolites pass out of the cell and into the blood in the same way.

When the metabolic needs of the tissues are low, parts of the capillary network can shut off, limiting blood flow. More blood is then available for those tissues with greater metabolic needs. Thus blood flow can be shunted in this way to areas that require a greater supply of oxygen and nutrients, e.g. exercising muscles.

Massage aids the dilation of these surface capillaries by reflex action, promoting blood flow. An accumulation of waste products in the tissues, or tension in muscle fibres, exert pressure on the capillaries and restrict blood flow. Massage helps to relieve this pressure as it speeds up the removal of waste products and promotes muscle relaxation. Thus the pressure is reduced and normal blood flow through the capillaries is restored. This helps the recovery of the muscles and restores normal function.

BLOOD

Blood is a viscous fluid (slightly sticky) which flows through the heart and blood vessels. It is composed of 55% plasma and 45% cells. (Plasma is a faintly yellow transparent fluid composed of 91% water, 7% proteins and 2% other solutes.) Its temperature is around 38°C and its pH is around 7.4 (slightly alkaline). The total volume of blood in the human body is 5–6 litres in men and 4–5 litres in women.

BLOOD CELLS

There are three main types of blood cell:

◆ **erythrocytes**: red blood cells which contain haemoglobin that transports oxygen and carbon dioxide

◆ **leucocytes**: white blood cells which protect the body against invading micro-organisms; they play a part in the body's defence system and immune reaction

◆ **thrombocytes** or **platelets**: they play an important role in blood clotting.

FUNCTIONS OF THE BLOOD

1 It **transports**

◆ oxygen from the lungs to body cells

◆ carbon dioxide from the cells to the lungs

◆ nutrients from the digestive tract to body cells

◆ metabolic waste products from cells to excretory organs

◆ hormones from endocrine glands to cells

◆ any drugs taken for medicinal purposes.

2 It **regulates**

◆ the water content of cells

◆ body heat, maintaining normal body temperature

◆ pH by means of buffers.

3 It **protects**

◆ against disease and infection by the action of leucocytes, which destroy micro-organisms through phagocytic action and production of antibodies

◆ against blood loss by the process of blood clotting.

BLOOD PRESSURE

This is the force or pressure which the blood exerts on the walls of the blood vessels. The blood pressure in arteries is higher than that in veins. Blood pressure varies with sex, age and weight, and with activities, stress levels or anxiety. The condition of the heart and vessels also affects pressure.

Normal average blood pressure rises to around 120 mmHg (millimetres of mercury) as the heart contracts (systolic pressure), and falls to around 80 mmHg as the heart relaxes (diastolic pressure). Blood pressure is measured using a **sphygmomanometer** and expressed as $BP = \dfrac{120}{80}$ mmHg.

PULSE

The pulse rate is the same as the heart rate, being around 74 beats per minute. The pulse can be felt in arteries because of the expansion and recoil of their walls during each ventricular contraction. The pulse is strongest in the arteries closest to the heart. The pulse is usually taken at the radial artery at the wrist, but can also be taken at the carotid artery in the neck and the brachial artery in the arm, medial to the biceps muscle.

EFFECTS OF MASSAGE ON BLOOD CIRCULATION

◆ Massage increases the blood flow through the area being treated, i.e. it produces hyperaemia (increased blood supply).

◆ It speeds up the flow of blood through the veins. Veins lie superficially (nearer the surface than arteries). As the hands move over the part in the direction of venous return, the blood is pushed along in the veins towards the heart. The deeper and faster the movements, the greater the flow. This venous blood carries away metabolic waste products more quickly. If these are allowed to accumulate in muscle tissue they produce pain and stiffness, and exert pressure which further restricts the circulation. Therefore, massage will relieve pain and stiffness by flushing out metabolic waste and relieving pressure on the capillaries which restores free flow of blood within the tissues.

◆ It increases the supply of fresh, oxygenated blood to the part. As the deoxygenated blood is moved along, the capillaries empty and fresh oxygenated blood flows into them more quickly. The nutrients and oxygen nourish the tissues and aid tissue recovery and repair.

◆ Massage dilates superficial arterioles and capillaries, which improves the exchange of substances in and out of cells via tissue fluid. This will improve the metabolic rate which, in turn, will improve the condition of the tissues. This dilation of the superficial capillaries produces an erythema (redness of the skin).

◆ Warmth is produced in the area due to the increased blood flow and friction of the hands on the part.

◆ Massage is thought to reduce the viscosity of the blood, reducing its rate of coagulation.

◆ Relaxing slow massage may reduce high blood pressure.

Lymphatic system

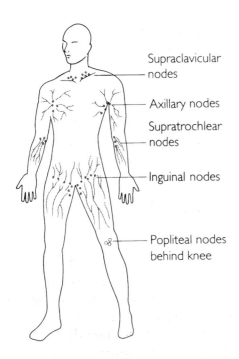

Supraclavicular nodes

Axillary nodes

Supratrochlear nodes

Inguinal nodes

Popliteal nodes behind knee

Figure 2.10 Lymphatic nodes of the body

The lymphatic system is closely associated with the cardio-vascular system and connects with it. The lymphatic system transports a fluid called lymph from the tissue spaces and returns it to the blood via the subclavian veins. It also transports fats in a fluid called **chyle** from the small intestine to the blood, and it plays an important role in protecting the body against infection.

The parts of the lymphatic system are:

◆ lymphatic capillaries, vessels and trunks: these are tubes which carry the fluid

◆ lymphatic nodes: arranged in groups throughout the body

◆ lymphatic organs: such as the spleen, thymus gland and tonsils

◆ lymphatic ducts: there are two ducts, the right lymphatic duct and the thoracic duct, which empty into the right and left subclavian veins

◆ lymph: the fluid flowing through the vessels.

Lymphatic capillaries begin as blind-end tubes forming a network among the tissue spaces. Their walls are very thin and allow fluid, larger proteins and particles to pass through. Because these larger particles and proteins are unable to pass through blood vessel walls, they are returned to the blood via the lymphatic system. These minute lymph capillaries then join together to form larger lymph vessels. Lymphatic vessels are very similar to veins in structure, but have thinner walls and a greater number of valves to prevent backward flow.

All lymph vessels drain into lymph nodes. These are strategically placed in groups along the path of the vessels. Many afferent vessels enter a node, but only one or two efferent vessels leave. Lymph nodes are small, bean-shaped structures up to 2 cm in length. Here the lymph is filtered, foreign substances are trapped and destroyed, and lymphocytes are produced which combat infection and disease. The efferent vessels leaving the nodes join to form lymph trunks. These empty into two main ducts:

1 **thoracic duct**: this receives lymph from the left arm, left side of the head and chest and all the body below the ribs; it empties into the left subclavian vein

2 **right lymphatic duct**: this receives lymph from the right upper quarter of the body, i.e. the right arm, right side of head and chest; it then empties into the right subclavian vein.

In this way the lymph is transported from the tissue spaces back to the blood. Any malfunction or blockage of the lymphatic system will result in swelling of the tissues known as **oedema**.

The speed at which lymph flows through the system depends on many factors, for example the contraction and relaxation of muscles help its return, as does negative pressure and movement of the chest during respiration. Exercise is therefore very important in aiding the flow of lymph. Areas of stasis and oedema can be improved by moving the joints and exercising the muscles of the swollen area. The volume of lymph passing into the capillaries and vessels depends on the pressure inside and outside the vessels.

Massage is very effective at speeding up the flow of lymph in the lymph vessels and thereby increasing the drainage of tissue fluid. Long effleurage strokes exert pressure and push the lymph along in the vessels towards the nearest set of lymph nodes (remember always move towards the nearest set of lymph nodes). The pressure (petrissage) manipulations squeeze the tissues. This pressure increases the amount of tissue fluid passing into the vessels to be drained away.

FUNCTIONS OF THE LYMPHATIC SYSTEM

1 The lymphatic system drains tissue fluid from the spaces between cells.

2 It transports this tissue fluid and proteins to

subclavian veins and so returns it back into the blood.

3 It transports fats from the small intestine to the blood.

4 It produces lymphocytes which protect and defend the body against infection and disease.

5 The nodes filter and remove broken down foreign substances and waste.

EFFECTS OF MASSAGE ON THE LYMPHATIC SYSTEM

◆ The flow of lymph in the lymph vessels is speeded up. As the hands move along in the direction of lymph drainage to the nearest group of lymph nodes, the speed of lymph flow is increased. Massage strokes should always be directed towards the nearest set of lymph nodes.

◆ Pressure on the tissues will facilitate the transfer of fluid across vessel walls. Fluid from the tissues will pass into the lymph vessels and will drain away more quickly; this will prevent or reduce oedema (swelling of the tissues).

◆ Larger particles of waste which are able to pass through the lymphatic vessel walls are removed more quickly.

The pressure and squeezing movements of petrissage are the most effective in reducing oedema, followed by effleurage. This effect is assisted if the part is elevated while being massaged, as gravity will assist drainage. Treatment of oedema using massage is described in Chapter 9.

Digestive system

The digestive system is concerned with the intake, breakdown and absorption of food substances. Carbohydrates, fats (lipids) and proteins are broken down into small molecules that can pass through the walls of the digestive tract into the bloodstream and then into body cells. Here they are used for energy, growth and repair of tissues.

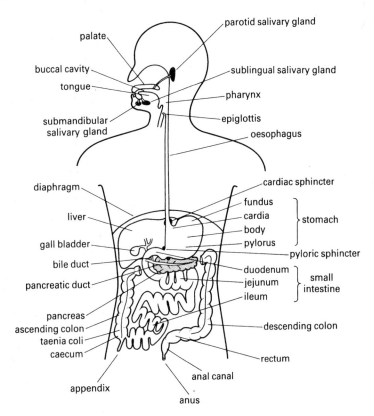

Figure 2.11 The digestive system

The digestive system is divisible into two main parts.

1 Gastro-intestinal tract or alimentary canal: this is a tube approximately 7 m in length. It starts at the mouth and ends at the anus. The parts of the gastro-intestinal tract are:

◆ mouth

◆ pharynx

◆ oesophagus

◆ stomach

◆ small intestine, divided into duodenum, jejunum and ileum

◆ large intestine, divided into caecum, colon, rectum and anal canal.

2 **Accessory structures** and organs connect with the tract and play an important role in the digestive process. They are:

◆ teeth

◆ tongue

◆ salivary glands

◆ gall-bladder

◆ pancreas.

◆ liver.

Substances move along the tract by a series of muscle contractions known as **peristalsis**. Massage stimulates peristalsis and also aids the movement through the tract.

PROCESS OF DIGESTION

The activities of the digestive system can be divided into four processes.

1 **Ingestion**: taking food into the body.

2 **Digestion**: the breaking down of food which involves two processes:

◆ mechanical breakdown by chewing and movements of the tract which churn the food

◆ chemical breakdown by enzymes secreted into the tract at various stages, e.g. saliva from salivary glands in the mouth; gastric juices in the stomach; pancreatic juice from the pancreas; bile from the gall-bladder; intestinal juice in the small intestine.

3 **Absorption**: the process by which digested food passes out of the tract into blood vessels and lymph capillaries and into cells.

4 **Elimination**: the passage of waste substances out of the body.

Effect of massage on the digestive system

◆ Abdominal massage stimulates peristalsis and the movement of digested food through the colon.

◆ Massage may be helpful to relieve constipation and flatulence.

Nervous system

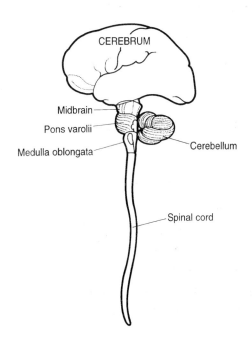

Figure 2.12 General view of the central nervous system

The nervous system is the communication and control system of the body. It works with the endocrine system to maintain homeostasis (body balance). The nervous system will sense changes, interpret them and initiate appropriate action. The nervous system is made up of:

◆ **central** nervous system, comprising the brain and spinal cord

◆ **peripheral** nervous system, comprising 12 pairs of cranial nerves arising from the brain and 31 pairs of spinal nerves arising from the spinal cord

◆ **autonomic** system.

The peripheral nerves carry impulses inwards from sensory receptors in sense organs to the brain. They also carry impulses from the brain to muscles and glands.

The autonomic system conducts information from the viscera to the central nervous system and information from the brain to smooth muscle, cardiac muscle and glands. This part is involuntary as it is not under conscious control.

During massage the sensory receptors in the skin convey impulses of touch and pressure to the central nervous system. If pressure is too light it can be irritating; if it is too deep or uneven it may be irritating or painful. Muscles then respond with increased tension. Slow, rhythmical, deep massage has a soothing effect on the nerve endings, promoting relaxation.

EFFECTS OF MASSAGE ON THE NERVOUS SYSTEM

◆ Slow, rhythmical massage produces a soothing, sedative effect on sensory nerve endings, promoting general relaxation.

◆ Vigorous brisk massage will have a stimulating effect, producing feelings of vigour and glow. Light hacking on either side of the vertebral column is particularly effective.

◆ If massage technique is poor or too heavy, the pain sensors in the skin will be stimulated. Painful manipulations will increase tension which is counter-productive and care must be taken to avoid this. Similarly, if movements are too light, i.e. barely touching the skin or tickling, this will have an irritating effect which will also increase tension and must be avoided.

Psychological effects of massage

The psychological effects of massage must also be considered.

◆ It creates feelings of well-being and health.

◆ It promotes feelings of vigour and increases energy.

◆ It increases postural awareness.

◆ It promotes feelings of being cared for and cosseted, which in turn promote relaxation, contentment and satisfaction.

◆ It reduces mental stress, which also enhances feelings of contentment and relaxation.

?

1 Give the organisational levels of the body.

2 Explain why it is important to identify skeletal bones prior to massaging an area.

3 Give two reasons why massage is used around joints.

4 State which massage movements are the most effective for stretching and freeing tight fascia around muscles.

5 Explain briefly why muscles may become stiff and painful following exercise and why massage will aid recovery.

6 State why warmth is created in the area being massaged.

7 Give two ways in which massage will aid desquamation.

8 Give the meaning of the following terms:
   (a) hyperaemia
   (b) erythema.

9 State two reasons why the skin will feel soft and supple after massage.

10 Explain how the circulation of blood to the area is increased by massage.

11 Name two groups of lymph nodes found in the leg and two found in the arm.

12 Explain briefly how massage prevents or relieves oedema.

13 Explain why massage is effective in relieving constipation.

14 Give three psychological effects of massage.

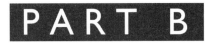

PART B

Consultation, preparation and massage movements

CHAPTER 3

Ethics and preparation

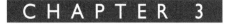

OBJECTIVES

After you have studied this chapter you will be able to:

1 explain what is meant by the term 'ethics'
2 list the factors which contribute to ethical behaviour
3 explain why safety and hygiene are important to the therapist
4 discuss the factors to consider when preparing the working area
5 prepare the working area
6 discuss the important factors to consider when selecting a massage couch
7 prepare a massage couch for treatment
8 discuss the procedure for preparing the working trolley
9 prepare the working trolley
10 explain the importance of having a selection of massage lubricants on the trolley
11 give the factors which contribute to high standards of personal hygiene
12 discuss the psychological preparation for massage
13 explain how you would prepare and position a client for massage
14 prepare and position a client for massage.

Ethics

Ethics refers to the standards and conduct of behaviour of an individual or professional group. Massage therapists must undergo a course of reputable training to enable them to acquire the understanding and skills necessary to carry out safe and effective treatment. In addition, they must consider their standard of behaviour in relation to colleagues, clients and the general public.

A high standard of ethical conduct will gain the confidence of clients and establish a sound reputation which is the basis for success. Always bear in mind the following points.

1 Look professional – be clean, neat and tidy.

2 Be punctual, keep appointments, do not cancel at the last minute. Always be on time for work.

3 Be discreet and refrain from gossip. Remember that clients often confide personal problems during consultation. These facts and all personal details must be treated with the utmost confidentiality. Do not repeat information or gossip to colleagues or others.

4 Be loyal to your employer and colleagues; create a friendly working relationship with all.

5 Be honest and reliable – this will gain the trust of others and establish a high reputation. Do not make false claims for treatments, but explain the benefits fairly. Be honest when advertising.

6 Speak correctly and politely to everyone. Do not use improper language. Consider the manner in which you answer or speak on the telephone.

7 Be polite and courteous at all times. There will be difficult clients to deal with – learn to handle tricky situations with tact and diplomacy.

8 Know and abide by local authority by-laws, rules and regulations for conducting your business.

9 Keep up to date with new theories, techniques and treatments. Attend courses on a regular basis and keep in touch with other professionals in your field.

10 Always practise the highest standards of personal and salon hygiene.

11 Do your utmost to deliver the most effective treatment suited to the needs of the client.

12 Organise yourself and your business to ensure a smooth-running, efficient service for the benefit of all concerned.

Preparation for massage

Preparation for massage involves the physical and mental preparation of the therapist and client as well as the preparation of the working area or room. The highest standards of hygiene and safety must be practised at all times. The massage therapist carries a heavy responsibility for protecting her/himself and the clients from the risk of cross-infection or any contamination by micro-organisms which cause disease. The therapist must be aware of, and practise, all the precautions and procedures necessary for protecting health and preventing the spread of disease.

PREPARATION OF WORKING AREA

◆ Ensure that the working area affords the client total privacy to change and receive treatment without being overlooked by others. The area may be a curtained section in a large salon, an individual walled cubicle or a small massage room. The therapist should ensure there is enough space to walk around the bed and work from all sides, and that there is room for a trolley with commodities and a stool.

◆ The area should be warm, well ventilated and draught free.

◆ It should be quiet, peaceful and free from distracting noise. Soft relaxing music may be played, but check with the client – some clients prefer to be quiet.

◆ The lighting should be soft and diffuse, not directed above the client and shining into her/his face.

◆ The colour scheme should be pale but warming, using pastel rather than harsh bold colours.

The above factors encourage relaxation which is of prime importance for massage treatments.

◆ The area must be spotlessly clean and tidy.

◆ Items required during the massage must be neatly arranged on the trolley shelf and protected with clean paper tissue or a small sheet.

◆ A plentiful supply of clean laundered towels and linen should be to hand.

◆ Extra pillows, small support pillows or rolled towels should also be to hand.

◆ Shower and toilet facilities for the client's use should be accessible and regularly cleaned.

◆ A hand basin or sink should be available for the therapist to wash her/his hands. Disposable towels or hot air dryers should be used to dry the hands. These must all be scrupulously clean.

◆ A lined bin should be to hand for disposal of waste.

☞ *Prepare a working area for massage.*

SELECTION OF MASSAGE COUCH

Selecting and purchasing a massage couch can be difficult as there is a wide choice available. Selection is often based on the cost of the couch, but there are other important points to bear in mind when buying. Consider the following points.

◆ It must be wide enough for the clients to turn over easily and to feel safe and secure.

◆ It must be long enough to support the length of the body.

◆ It must be robust, secure and firm. It must not move or rock with the massage nor grate or squeak as this will disturb the client and prevent her/him from relaxing.

◆ It must be at the correct height for working. If it is too high the therapist will have to stretch to reach certain areas. S/he will not be able to use body weight correctly to apply the required pressure. If it is too low the therapist will have to bend over too much. This will cause shoulder and back problems. When standing upright next to the couch with the arms by the side, the couch should be just below the level of the wrist.

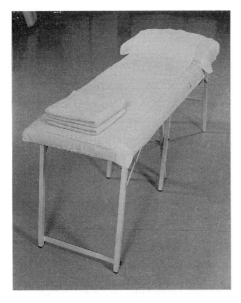

Figure 3.1 A prepared massage couch

- The covering should be of smooth, washable material which is easy to wipe over and keep clean.

- If you need a couch that you can move from room to room or take on home visits then select the portable folding variety. Ensure that the legs are sturdy and that the hinges are secure and firm. Apply pressure sideways and to the top and bottom to test whether it shakes, rocks or stays firm.

If you are using the couch for other treatments, select from the multi-purpose varieties. The most useful couches are the adjustable height hydraulic varieties, but these are expensive and may be outside your budget. However, they are ideal for massage as the height can be adjusted to accommodate all types of client such as small and thin or large and obese. Some couches have a hole for the nose and mouth, to make positioning and breathing easier when lying prone.

PREPARATION OF MASSAGE COUCH

Prepare the couch before the client arrives.

- Cover the entire surface with a towelling or cotton sheet – the fitted types are best as they stay neat and tidy.

- Next cover this with a large bath towel or cotton sheet. This must be removed and boil washed after each client and a clean one re-applied. Many salons and colleges use disposable paper sheets (bed roll) to save on the laundry – these are quite acceptable, but they can tear and crumple during the massage and may interfere with some movements.

- Use one or two pillows for the head. Cover these with pillow slips and then a towel.

- Fold two large towels and place them at the foot of the bed. These will be used to cover the client.

- Place extra pillows, large and small, and a rolled towel on the trolley for use if extra support is required during the massage.

Collect information from advertising leaflets on a variety of massage couches and select one that you feel would be suitable for you, giving reasons for your selection.

PREPARATION OF TROLLEY OR TABLE

◆ Select a trolley or table with a hard, smooth surface, free of cracks and easy to clean. Ensure that it is robust and sturdy so that it cannot be pushed over. Wheels are an advantage as the trolley may be pulled or pushed into a convenient position.

◆ Place the trolley near the massage couch so that all items will be to hand when required.

◆ Wipe the shelves with disinfectant of the correct dilution.

◆ Cover the shelves with paper sheets – fold under all edges for neatness.

◆ Arrange cleaned bottles and bowls neatly on this sheet. Always place commodities in the same order to ensure that they are easy to identify and reach when needed. Plastic baskets may be used to hold the bottles neatly. Clean these with disinfectant before loading.

◆ The following items should be laid out on the top shelf of the trolley:

(a) a bottle of cologne – for cleaning the skin if the client has not taken a shower
(b) a bottle of surgical spirit – to clean the feet
(c) a good quality oil or cream – used as a medium for the massage
(d) talcum powder or corn starch – these powders may be used instead of oil or cream as a massage medium. They work well for very hairy clients
(e) a bowl containing tissues and balls of cotton wool
(f) a bowl for placing the client's jewellery is sometimes used, but it is much safer to ask the client to place jewellery in her bag and place this under the couch.

◆ A bowl for waste, lined with clean disposable tissue, should be placed on a lower shelf, *or* a bin with disposable liner may be placed under the trolley. This is to avoid the risk of contamination of the commodities.

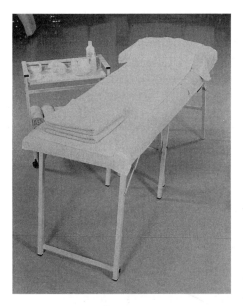

Figure 3.2 A prepared massage trolley

◆ Cover the shelf and commodities with a clean paper sheet when not in use. This will protect items from dust and dirt.

◆ At the end of each day, strip the trolley down. Wipe the shelves with disinfectant, clean all the bottles and bowls, then either store the commodities in a cupboard ready for use the following day or re-lay the trolley and cover.

Clean a trolley or table and prepare it for massage.

SELECTION OF OILS AND CREAMS

There are a wide variety of oils and creams available. Selection will depend largely on personal choice regarding cost, viscosity and the perfume used. Clients sometimes develop allergies to certain oils and creams, so it is important to have alternatives to hand. Itching, intense erythema, heat, papules or pustles all indicate sensitivity and the oil or cream must be changed. Always select narrow-necked bottles or tubes with small apertures, or preferably self-dispensing plunge types. A small opening is essential as it reduces the risk of contamination by micro-organisms.

PREPARATION OF THERAPIST

Before carrying out a massage therapists must prepare themselves physically, paying due consideration to high standards of professionalism and hygiene. They must also prepare psychologically and give due thought to the type of massage required.

PERSONAL HYGIENE

◆ A daily bath or shower should be taken to maintain cleanliness of the skin, hair and nails, and to remove stale sweat odours.

◆ An antiperspirant should be used to prevent excessive sweating and the odour of stale sweat.

◆ Hair should be clean and neat; it should be kept short or tied back from the face. Hair must never fall forward around the therapist's face and shoulders or touch the client.

◆ Nails must be well manicured and kept short; nails should not protrude above the fleshy part of the finger tip. Massage movements cannot be correctly performed if the nails are long, and long nails may harbour dirt or bacteria. Nail enamel should not be worn as some clients may be sensitive to the product and an allergic reaction may result.

◆ Hands must be well cared for; they must be smooth and warm for massage. Therapists should protect the hands with rubber gloves when doing chores. A good quality hand lotion should be used night and morning. Gloves should be worn in cold weather. Therapists should not massage with cuts or abrasions on the hands.

◆ Jewellery should be removed or kept to a minimum of wedding ring and small ear studs. Rings, bracelets and watches can harbour micro-organisms or can injure the client if dragged on the skin. Long earrings and necklaces may jangle, producing a noise which is disturbing to the client.

◆ Underwear and tights should be changed daily and washed in hot soapy water.

◆ White, short-sleeved overalls should be crisp, well laundered and changed frequently (e.g. every other day). The style should allow free unrestricted movement of the arms during massage.

◆ Feet should be well cared for and washed and dried thoroughly once a day, using foot powder if necessary. A clean pair of tights should be worn each day; support tights will help prevent tired legs and varicose veins. Well fitting low-heeled or flat shoes without holes or peeptoes will protect the feet and avoid pressure points.

◆ Working uniform should not be worn out of the salon. Outdoor clothing worn to work should be changed in a cloakroom to prevent micro-organisms being brought into the salon.

◆ Therapists suffering from colds and infections should not treat clients if possible, but the wearing of a surgical mask will greatly reduce the risk of cross-infection.

◆ Therapists must wash their hands before touching a client and after cleaning the feet prior to the massage.

PSYCHOLOGICAL PREPARATION

Preparing the mind enhances concentration and co-ordination and contributes to expertise and effectiveness of the massage.

◆ Develop a calm, tranquil but positive attitude. It is important to feel secure, confident and relaxed yourself as this is transmitted to the client both by your attitude and through your hands.

◆ Develop co-ordination between mind and body. The hands and body must move as a whole – think of your foot position, posture, arm/hand positions, speed, pressure and rhythm. Remember that massage is a skill which must be learned and requires constant practice to perform it well. It is very similar to learning to play a musical instrument.

◆ Develop sensory awareness, i.e. the ability to sense and visualise structures through the hands. Through the sensory receptors in the hands you learn to identify bony points, degrees of tone or tension in muscles, and variations found on different tissues and different clients. This ability only comes through practice and the experience of treating a variety of different types of client, e.g. young, old, thin, obese, well toned, poorly toned, tense or relaxed.

◆ Learn to synchronise speed, rhythm and depth so that these remain consistent throughout the treatment. These will vary depending on the effects required (see page 111). Maximum effectiveness of the treatment will occur only if these factors are co-ordinated.

PREPARATION OF CLIENT

◆ Speak to the client in a polite and friendly manner.

◆ Maintain client privacy at all times.

◆ Take the client's outdoor clothes or show her/him where to hang them.

◆ Show the client the treatment area and shower room.

◆ Ask the client to undress and give her/him a robe or towel to wear.

◆ Ask the client to remove all jewellery and place it in a bag for safe keeping.

◆ Instruct the client how to use the shower.

◆ Bring the client back to the treatment area.

◆ Carry out a client consultation and discuss the treatment (see Chapter 4).

◆ Explain fully and ask if the client has any queries.

◆ If the client has long hair, ask her/him to tie it up or provide a protective cover.

LYING

◆ Help the client onto the couch.

◆ Position the client correctly on the couch. A correct, well-supported position will ensure that the client is comfortable and will aid muscle relaxation. If the client is not well supported and comfortable, the muscles will be tense and will contract to hold the body parts. S/he will become restless and unable to relax and the massage will be ineffective. The position of the client must also allow the therapist to reach all areas easily without stooping or over-stretching.

◆ Ask the client to lie centrally on the bed.

◆ Ensure that the client's body is straight.

◆ In the **supine** lying position (on the back) offer the client one or two pillows under the head for support. Another pillow placed under the knees will help to flatten the lumbar spine. Some clients like this knee support and it is particularly beneficial for those with back pain. This pillow must be fairly small and firm so that it does not hinder the leg massage.

◆ In the **prone** lying position (face down) the head is

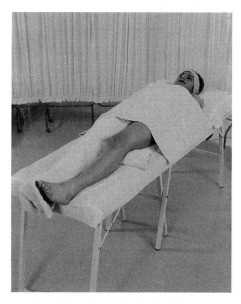

Figure 3.3 Positioning client for massage (a) supine

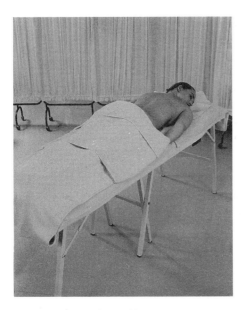

Figure 3.3 (b) prone

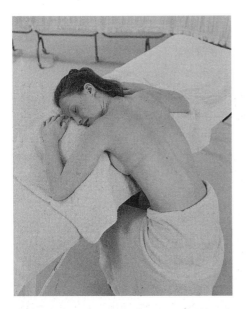

Figure 3.3 (c) sitting

usually turned to one side, with or without a pillow under the head depending on client preference. A pillow placed under the abdomen will round out the lumbar spine which will make those clients with lordosis more comfortable. A small firm pad or tightly rolled towel can be placed under the ankles. This ensures that the anterior tibial tendons are not over-stretched. Alternatively the feet may just hang over the edge of the bed. The arms may be placed down along the body or bent and placed on either side of the head.

◆ Cover the client with two towels: one placed across the upper trunk from neck to waist; the other placed lengthways from the waist to the feet.

◆ Each part is uncovered when being worked on and then re-covered as the massage moves on.

◆ Always ask if the client is warm and comfortable.

SITTING

Massage of the neck and upper back is frequently done with the client sitting. It is also a comfortable position for the pregnant client requiring massage for low back pain.

◆ Place a stool to the side or the end of a couch or table. Cover with a towel.

◆ Place one or two pillows on the couch and cover with a towel.

◆ Ask the client to undress, sit on the stool and lean forward onto the pillows.

◆ Ensure that the client is comfortable and well supported, with the arms and head resting on the pillow.

◆ Cover with a towel until the massage begins.

 Role play with a friend as the client.

(a) Position the client on the couch and prepare her/him for massage of the back.

(b) Position the client for a neck and upper back massage. Ensure her/his comfort at all times.

USE OF HEAT PRIOR TO MASSAGE

Heating the tissues prior to massage enhances the effect of the massage. The application of heat will dilate the superficial blood vessels, and increase the circulation and metabolic rate. The warmth will relieve pain and tension, thus promoting relaxation. These factors will increase the effect of the massage which follows.

◆ Mild gentle heat may be given for 15–20 minutes.

◆ Any form of heating may be used, depending on client preference, suitability and availability; for example, infra red, radiant heat, steam bath, sauna bath, hot pack, etc.

◆ Heat should not be used if contra-indicated, nor in the treatment of oedema or acute injury.

(The principles of heat treatments can be found in *Body Therapy and Facial Work*, 1994, Mo Rosser, Hodder & Stoughton).

?

1 Explain briefly why high ethical standards are required in a massage therapist.

2 List ten factors which contribute to ethical behaviour.

3 State briefly how you would deal with a difficult client.

4 List the important factors which ensure high standards of personal hygiene.

5 Explain why the therapist's nails should be short and free of nail enamel.

6 Explain why outdoor clothing should not be worn in the treatment area.

7 Discuss the importance of psychological preparation prior to massage.

8 List the important factors to consider when preparing the massage area.

9 Explain why the lighting in the working area should be soft and unobtrusive.

10 Give the factors that you would consider when purchasing a massage couch.

11 Explain how you would prepare the couch for massage.

12 List the items that must be arranged on the trolley prior to massage.

13 State why it is important to have a selection of oils and creams available.

14 Give the factors that must be considered when positioning the client on the couch.

15 Explain how you would position a client with lordosis to ensure maximum comfort.

16 Explain how you would position a client for massage to the neck and upper back.

CHAPTER 4

Client consultation

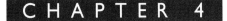

OBJECTIVES

After you have studied this chapter you will be able to:

1 discuss the importance and purpose of detailed consultation
2 carry out a detailed consultation
3 list the essential information required on a record card
4 design a record card for use in massage
5 list the contra-indications to massage
6 recognise the conditions where medical advice must be sought
7 identify conditions where extra care must be taken.

Initial consultation

The consultation is a very important part of the treatment – sufficient time must be allowed so that it is not rushed.

The initial consultation will provide detailed information which must be accurately recorded on a treatment card. This must be filed in a safe and accessible place and used each time the client attends for treatment. Before subsequent treatments, a brief consultation is usually sufficient to establish the effects and outcomes of the previous treatments and whether any changes are to be made or further action is to be taken.

For the consultation the client should be seated comfortably, with the therapist positioned alongside or opposite. The environment should feel warm and private.

Detailed consultation is important for the following reasons:

- to establish a rapport with the client and put her/him at ease

- to develop mutual trust and gain the client's confidence

- to gain information on the client's past and present state of mental and physical health

- to identify any contra-indications

- to gain insight into the client's lifestyle, responsibilities, work environment, leisure activities, etc.

- to identify any particular needs and expectations of the treatment

- to establish the most appropriate form of treatment and to discuss and agree this with the client

- to fully explain the treatment to the client, including the procedure, expected effects, timing and frequency

- to agree a treatment plan and cost with the client so that s/he fully understands the financial commitment

- to answer queries and questions related to the treatment and to allay doubts and fears.

The information gathered will provide a baseline from which the appropriate treatment is planned, the effectiveness of the treatment can be judged and any necessary changes or adjustments made.

Note: all the information given must be treated in confidence.

ESSENTIAL INFORMATION

The following personal, medical and environmental factors should be recorded on the consultation card.

Personal details

- status

- name

- address

- date of birth
- home and work telephone numbers
- occupation
- doctor's name, address and telephone number

Past medical history

- surgical operations
- pregnancies
- serious illness

Present medical history

- medication
- general health
- current treatments
- identification of stress: work, home or other sources

Massage analysis

- contra-indications
- has client received massage in the past?
- how long ago?
- number of sessions
- did client benefit from the massage?
- reasons for requesting massage

Examination

- posture
- height
- weight
- skin type: smooth/supple; dry/flaky; loose/stretched
- stretch marks
- areas of hard fat/cellulite

- areas of soft fat

- general muscle tone

- bony protuberances

- fluid retention

- disfiguration or distortion of surface anatomy

- other factors which may affect massage

Ask the client to read and sign the completed record card.

Contra-indications to massage

A contra-indication is a condition which, if present, means that the treatment should not be carried out. Massage should not be given if any of the following conditions are present:

- **skin diseases or disorders**: these may be irritated or spread by the friction of the hands over the part or by the lubricant, e.g. eczema, psoriasis, acne, any skin infections

- **cuts and abrasions**: risk of infection and blood contamination

- **recent or extensive bruising**: small bruises can be avoided

- **recent haemorrhage** or bleeding

- **recent scar tissue**: there is a danger of breaking down recently formed scar tissue. However, when the scar is completely healed (after about six months) massage may be given and is useful for stretching and loosening old contracted scar tissue

- **recent operations**

- **sunburn or wind burn** on the area to be massaged

- **large, lumpy or inflamed moles**: other areas may be massaged

- **warts or skin tags**: avoid these

- **bone fractures**: avoid until healing is complete; other areas may be massaged

- **metal pins or plates** inserted to support fractured bones: avoid the area

- **swollen, hot or painful joints**

- **recent sprains or muscle strains**: there may be damage to ligaments, tendons and muscle fibres; these must be allowed to heal before massage

- **any swellings, painful or inflamed areas of unknown origin**: massage is used to prevent or alleviate oedema (swelling in the tissues), but medical advice must be sought if there is doubt as to the cause of the oedema and whether massage is suitable

- **heart conditions**: because massage affects the rate of blood flow it may have an undesirable effect if there is a heart condition. Always seek medical advice if a client has heart problems. Stress-related heart problems may be helped by relaxing massage

- **high blood pressure**: although blood pressure varies with age, weight and fitness, some people have consistently high blood pressure. Medical advice should be obtained if such people request massage. Massage can frequently help, especially if the condition is stress related

- **low blood pressure**: again medical advice should be obtained before massage treatment is given. These clients may feel dizzy or faint if they sit up or get off the bed too quickly following treatment. Always supervise and give assistance if necessary.

- **thrombosis**: this is a blood clot in the veins; massage may disturb and dislodge the clot from the vein wall so that it travels through the veins and could cause a blockage in a vital organ such as the lungs or brain, with very serious consequences. Thrombosis is quite common in the deep veins of the calf. Anyone with pain in the calf should be referred to their doctor

- **phlebitis**: inflammation of the lining of the vein which is often present with thrombosis and should be referred in the same way

- **history of embolism**: blood clot circulating in the blood stream

- **varicose veins**: any obvious, protruding varicose veins must be avoided. Massage proximal to the veins can help relieve the pressure

- **weak muscles with poor tone**: effleurage and gentle kneading movements may be used but wringing and all percussion movements must be avoided

- **spastic muscles** (i.e. muscle with increased tone): massage may increase spasticity and must be avoided

- **dysfunction or disorders to the nervous system**: such as multiple sclerosis, strokes, Parkinson's disease, etc.

- **cancer**: any history of cancer, as it can spread via the lymphatic system

- **epilepsy**: it is safe to massage controlled epilepsy, but always seek medical consent. Do not leave anyone suffering from epilepsy unattended in a cubicle or on the couch

- **diabetes**: some sufferers can be treated but as tissue healing is impaired in these clients, great care must be taken not to damage tissues particularly of the lower leg and foot. Seek medical advice before treating.

Old clients with thin, crêpey skin and poor muscle tone must be massaged with great care. Pressure should be kept light to moderate and plenty of lubrication must be applied to prevent further stretching the skin. All percussion movements, i.e. hacking, cupping, beating and pounding, should not be given.

If massage is contra-indicated tell the client gently, explain carefully and do not alarm her/him. Tell the client that it is for her/his own protection and that you will continue treatment when the condition has cleared or when medical consent is given.

> *Compile a neat, clearly worked consultation card for use in the salon for massage clients.*

Referring clients to a medical practitioner

Doctors are very busy people and do not have time to write letters in response to queries from therapists. It is therefore a good idea to compose a standard letter which explains the facts clearly and merely requires the doctor's signature. An example (for a female client) is provided on page 71.

?

1 Give the meaning of the term 'contra-indication'.

2 List the reasons for the importance of a detailed consultation.

3 Name two contra-indications where medical advice should be sought.

4 Name two conditions where extra care should be taken.

5 Explain the factors you would consider when conducting an examination of a client prior to massage.

Address of salon

Date

Doctor's address

Dear Dr [name]

Your patient, [name], of [address], has requested a [type of massage, e.g. general body massage] once a week. During my consultation with her, she mentioned that she has been suffering from [illness, e.g. diabetes] for some years. I would be very grateful if you would indicate her suitability for treatment by signing the consent below.

Thank you.

Yours faithfully

[Your name]

....

Doctor's consent

I agree that the massage treatment you suggest would be suitable for this patient.

Signed

....

[Doctor's signature]

CHAPTER 5

Classification of massage and the effleurage group

After you have studied this chapter you will be able to:

1 list the four main groups of massage
2 list the manipulations that belong to each group
3 explain the differences between effleurage and stroking
4 describe the techniques of effleurage and stroking
5 explain the effects of effleurage and stroking
6 explain when these manipulations may be used
7 perform effleurage manipulations on a client's back or leg
8 perform stroking on a client's back or leg
9 adapt effleurage to suit a variety of clients and conditons.

Classification of massage movements

The terminology used to describe and group massage movements has evolved over the centuries. There are differences in terminology from country to country and from school to school. The terminology used today is based on the Swedish remedial massage devised in Sweden by the physiologist Per Henrik Ling, and Dr Johann Mezgner of Holland. This has been modified over the years with input from French, German and British physicians and practitioners.

The names of the groups describe the action of the hands on the tissues. The four main groups are:

1 **effleurage**: where the hands skim over the surface of the tissues

2 **petrissage**: where the hands press down or lift and squeeze the tissues

3 **percussion or tapotement**: where the hands strike the tissues

4 **vibrations**: where the hands vibrate or shake the tissues.

Each of these groups may be further broken down into different manipulations which have their own technique and specific effects.

Table 5.1 Classification of massage movements

Group	Manipulations
Effleurage	Effleurage
	Stroking
Petrissage	Kneading
	Wringing
	Picking up
	Skin rolling or muscle rolling
	Frictions – circular or transverse
Percussion or tapotement	Hacking
	Cupping or clapping
	Beating
	Pounding
Vibrations	Vibrations
	Shaking

Effleurage group

The word 'effleurage' comes from the French verb *effleurer* which means 'to skim over'. There are two manipulations within this group:

1 effleurage

2 stroking.

Although the two manipulations are similar, in that the relaxed hands move over the surface of the body, there are important differences to note. These differences lie in the direction of the strokes and in the differences in the pressure applied.

DIFFERENCES BETWEEN EFFLEURAGE AND STROKING

◆ Effleurage must always follow the direction of venous return back to the heart and the direction of lymphatic drainage towards the nearest group of lymph nodes. Stroking may be performed in any direction.

◆ The pressure during effleurage may be light, moderate or heavy, but always increases at the end of the stroke towards the lymph nodes. The pressure of stroking is selected at the commencement and is maintained throughout. It also may be light, moderate or heavy pressure depending on the type of massage given.

◆ When performing effleurage, hand contact is maintained during the return of the stroke, although little pressure is applied. When performing stroking, the hands may maintain contact or may lift off the part on return.

Effleurage

As previously explained, effleurage is a manipulation where one or both hands move over the surface of the body, applying varying degrees of pressure according to the type of massage being given. Effleurage will produce superficial effects when the pressure is light to moderate, but will produce deeper effects if the pressure is heavy.

TECHNIQUE

1 Ensure that the client is warm and comfortable.

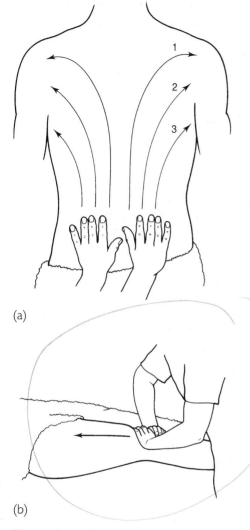

(a)

(b)

Figure 5.1 Effleurage (a) on back (b) on thigh

2 Take up a walk standing position with the outside foot forward: make sure you can reach all parts.

3 Remember to bend the front knee as the movement progresses and use body weight to apply pressure (pressure must not be applied through the arms and shoulders alone). Keep your back straight.

4 Ensure that your hands are warm, relaxed and supple – they must mould and adapt to the body contours.

5 The hands must move in the direction of venous return back to the heart, beginning distally and working proximally.

6 The strokes must be directed towards, and end at, a group of lymph nodes wherever possible.

7 The pressure should increase slightly at the end of the stroke.

8 The hands maintain contact on the return of stroke but apply little pressure.

9 The movement must be smooth and rhythmical, with continuous flow and even pressure.

10 The whole of the palmar surface of the hand, fingers and thumb should maintain contact with the body in a relaxed manner. (Do not extend, abduct or link the thumbs, and do not spread the fingers out as these habits will give uneven pressure.)

11 The hands usually work together with even pressure and rhythm. However, the hands may be used alternately when care must be taken to maintain an even pressure under each hand and to synchronise the flow and rhythm.

12 On small areas, one hand may work while the other supports the tissues. On very small areas such as the face, fingers or toes, the thumbs only may be used in a sweeping action.

ADAPTING EFFLEURAGE

◆ Effleurage must be adapted to suit the client and the

objectives of the treatment. For example, on the older thin client with poor muscle tone, the pressure will be light to moderate and plenty of oil will be applied. On a younger or fitter and well-toned client, the pressure can be deeper. A good covering of adipose tissue can take deeper pressure.

♦ For a relaxing massage, the effleurage will be rhythmical, slow and of medium depth. For a stimulating or vigorous massage, the effleurage will be rhythmical but faster and deeper.

♦ The effleurage performed at the end, to complete the treatment, should become progressively slower.

♦ When treating oedema, effleurage will *follow* kneading and squeezing movements – not precede them as is usual. The strokes will also change to begin proximally near the lymph nodes and work distally.

♦ When treating areas of cellulite the heavier movements of kneading and percussion are interspersed with effleurage, and the treatment ends with effleurage to increase drainage.

EFFECTS

1 As the hands press on the tissues and move along they push the blood in the veins onwards. This speeds up the removal of deoxygenated blood and waste products from the tissues. Deep effleurage performed over muscles after exercise or any athletic performance will thus hasten the removal of lactic acid and relieve pain and stiffness. Effleurage will help the muscle to recover and return to normal function.

2 As a result of increased venous drainage the blood flow through the capillary beds is speeded up. This increases the arterial blood flow, bringing oxygen and nutrients to the tissues more quickly. These factors improve the condition of the tissues.

3 The increased blood flow will increase the metabolic rate of the tissue cells which also will improve their condition.

4 The increased blood flow and friction of the hands

on the part will warm the area. This will aid relaxation and relieve pain.

5 The flow of lymph in the lymphatic vessels is also speeded up as the hands move along. This is directed towards the lymph nodes where it is filtered and then drained into larger vessels. Lymph removes large protein particles and tissue fluid from tissue spaces. Speeding up the drainage prevents stagnation of fluid in the tissues which would result in oedema (swelling of the tissues). Effleurage and squeezing are manipulations used in the treatment of oedema.

6 The increased blood flow and dilation of capillaries in the skin will produce an erythema which improves skin tone. The increased blood flow also nourishes the skin, improving its condition.

7 The cells of the stratum basale are stimulated and mitosis (cell division) increases. As more cells are produced they move upwards to the surface, improving the condition of the skin.

8 The movement and friction of the hands over the skin removes the dry flaking cells of the stratum corneum – thus desquamation is speeded up and the condition of the skin improves.

9 The oil or cream used as a medium nourishes and improves the skin.

10 The sebaceous glands are stimulated and produce more sebum, which keeps the skin soft and supple.

11 The warmth generated by massage stimulates the sweat glands, increasing the elimination of waste products.

12 Slow rhythmical effleurage has a soothing effect on sensory nerve endings in the skin which will promote relaxation. However, if the pressure is very light or barely touching, the nerve endings will be irritated, or if the pressure is very deep the pain sensors will be stimulated. Both these effects will increase tension and should be avoided.

USES

Effleurage is used:

1 to stimulate venous drainage and a sluggish circulation (to prevent varicose veins and varicose ulcers)

2 to stimulate lymphatic drainage and prevent or relieve oedema

3 to improve the condition of muscle tissue

4 to improve the condition and suppleness of the skin and produce an erythema

5 to promote relaxation using rhythmical slow movements of medium depth

6 to invigorate an area using rhythmical, fast movements with deep pressure

7 to remove waste products of fatigue following exercise, sport or athletic performance, thus relieving pain and promoting quick recovery

8 to help the warm-up of muscles prior to athletic performance (this must be used in addition, not instead of, a set of warm-up and stretch exercises). Warm-up exercise must always be performed prior to exercise sessions or athletic performance

9 as the first manipulation to enable the client to become accustomed to the therapist's hands and to aid client relaxation; as the last manipulation to conclude the massage.

10 as a linkage movement to provide continuity and smooth transition between other massage groups

11 to spread the oil or cream used as the massage medium.

Stroking

Stroking is very similar to effleurage in that one or both hands move over the surface of the body applying varying degrees of pressure, but there are differences as previously explained.

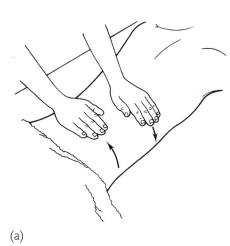

(a)

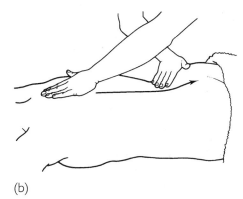

(b)

Figure 5.2 Stroking (a) across back (b) down erector spine

TECHNIQUE

1 The therapist's stance depends on the direction of movement – walk standing (one foot in front of the other) if working top to bottom, stride standing (feet apart) if working from side to side.

2 The hands must be warm, relaxed and supple; they may mould and adapt to the contours of the body but this is not always so.

3 The wrists must be very flexible and loose.

4 The movement can be performed in any direction.

5 The pressure is selected at the commencement of the stroke and maintained throughout the stroke. This pressure may be light to moderate for a relaxing massage or firm and heavy for a vigorous massage.

6 The movements must be rhythmical with continuous flow.

7 The hands may or may not be lifted off the part at the end of the stroke.

8 The whole of the palmar surface of the hand, fingers and thumb may remain in contact with the part or the fingers only may be used.

9 The hands usually work alternately, one hand commencing a stroke as the other reaches the end.

10 The hands may work in opposite directions if working across the back, one beginning on the right side, the other on the left side, then crossing the back. Stroking is frequently performed from the nape of the neck to the base of the spine, or transversely across the abdomen, back or thigh.

EFFECTS

Soothing stroking, performed slowly with light pressure:

1 soothes sensory nerve endings in the skin which promotes relaxation

2 produces contraction of superficial capillaries which will cool down an area

3 produces feelings of deep relaxation which may induce sleep and help insomnia.

Stimulating stroking, performed vigorously with pressure:

1 stimulates sensory nerve endings which counteracts feelings of lethargy and tiredness

2 produces dilation of superficial capillaries which increases the circulation to the skin, giving an erythema

3 stimulates the sebaceous glands to secrete more sebum, which keeps the skin soft and supple, and the sweat glands to produce more sweat

4 may stimulate peristalsis and general movement of the contents of the colon. Use deep digital stroking of the abdomen in the direction of the colon.

USES

Soothing stroking is used:

1 to soothe and relax a tense, nervous client

2 to help insomnia and promote sleep

3 to produce vasoconstriction on a hot, oedematous area.

Stimulating stroking is used:

1 to stimulate a lethargic client and arouse a tired one

2 to produce an erythema and warm up an area

3 over the abdomen to prevent or treat constipation.

Role play the following with a partner:

◆ practise effleurage and stroking on each other

◆ comment on depth, speed, rhythm, continuity

◆ adapt effleurage for a relaxing massage, i.e. slow, deep, rhythmical

◆ adapt effleurage for a vigorous, stimulating massage, i.e. fast, deep, rhythmical

◆ always consider stance, posture and continuity.

?

1 List the four main groups of massage.

2 List the movements (manipulations) in each group.

3 Give three different points of technique between stroking and effleurage.

4 Explain how you would adapt effleurage movements for the following clients:

   (a) the older, thin client

   (b) the young, fit, well-toned client.

5 Give six effects of effleurage.

6 List four uses of effleurage.

7 List six effects of stroking.

8 Give four conditions which would benefit from stroking.

9 Explain why the pressure of effleurage strokes should always be towards the heart.

10 Explain how effleurage strokes are adapted when treating oedema.

CHAPTER 6

Petrissage group

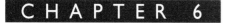

After you have studied this chapter you will be able to:

1 list the five manipulations that belong to this group
2 subdivide and list all forms of kneading
3 describe the technique for each manipulation
4 explain the effects of each manipulation
5 explain the uses of each manipulation
6 identify manipulations for use on specific areas of the body
7 perform each manipulation on specified areas of the body.

The word 'petrissage' comes from the French verb *pétrir* meaning 'to knead'. There are five manipulations in this group, but some can be further subdivided:

1 kneading

2 wringing

3 picking up

4 skin and muscle rolling

5 frictions.

All the manipulations in this group apply pressure to the tissues, but each manipulation differs in technique. The true kneading manipulations apply pressure to the tisssue and move them over underlying bone in a circular movement. However, other manipulations have evolved where the tissues are lifted away from the bone, squeezed and then released. Some of the manipulations in this group are quite difficult to perform and much practice is needed to perfect them.

Kneading

There are many forms of kneading. The terminology used for each one will tell you what should be done, so study them carefully.

◆ **Palmar kneading**: this is kneading with the palmar surface of the hand. There are different forms of palmar kneading.

◆ **Digital kneading**: this is kneading with the digits (i.e. the fingers) – the index, middle and ring fingers are usually used.

◆ **Thumb kneading**: this is kneading with the thumbs.

◆ **Ulnar border kneading**: this is kneading with the ulnar border of the hand (ulnar bone or little finger side).

PALMAR KNEADING

Palmar kneading applies pressure to the tissues through the palmar surface of the hands and fingers, and moves the superficial tissues over the deep tissues.

The hands work in a circular motion, applying pressure on the upward part of the circle. This ensures that the pressure is applied in the direction of venous return to the heart and lymphatic drainage to the lymph nodes.

A variety of methods of palmar kneading may be used – selection depends on the area being treated.

◆ **Single-handed kneading**: one hand performs the kneading while the other supports the tissues on the other side. This is useful on smaller muscles such as triceps and biceps in the arm.

◆ **Alternate palmar kneading**: one hand works slightly before the other, resulting in alternate upward pressure. The hands are placed on either side of a limb (e.g. one on the abductors and one on the adductors of the leg) or they may be placed on the right and left side of the spine if kneading the back from the nape of the neck to the sacrum. One hand

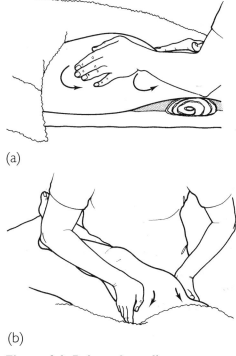

(a)

(b)

**Figure 6.1 Palmar kneading
(a) single-handed kneading
(b) alternate palmar kneading**

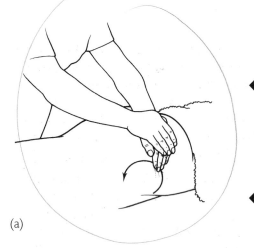

(a)

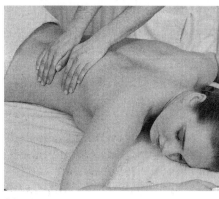

(b)

Figure 6.2 Palmar kneading
(a) reinforced palmar kneading
(b) double-handed kneading

starts, then after half a circle the other hand begins producing alternate pressure upwards. This produces excellent mobilisation of the tissues.

◆ **Reinforced palmar kneading**: one hand lies directly on top of the other, reinforcing its movement. This produces very deep pressure which is useful on large muscle groups, such as the quadriceps, hamstrings, posterior tibials, and also on areas of dense adipose tissue over the hips, waist and sides of the trunk.

◆ **Double-handed kneading**: the hands work side by side, moving the tissues in a large circle with the pressure upwards. This is useful when covering large areas, e.g. from one side of the back to the other. It is also used over the quadriceps and hamstrings on very large thighs.

Although these manipulations have different names according to the way the hands work, they are all methods of palmar kneading and the basic technique is the same for all.

TECHNIQUE

1 Stand in walk or stride standing, depending on the direction of work.

2 The hands must be warm, relaxed and supple – they must mould to the contours of the body.

3 The pressure must be directed upwards through the palms and fingers in the direction of venous return to the heart and the lymphatic drainage.

4 The pressure is applied upwards on each half circle and then released slightly to complete the circle.

5 The pressure must be firm enough to prevent skin rubbing. The flesh should move under the hands.

6 The heel of the hand must not dig into the part.

7 The movements must be smooth, rhythmical and with continuous flow.

8 The hands may work upwards and downwards in continuous sequence, or they may work in one direction and slide back, maintaining contact.

EFFECTS

1 The alternate pressure and relaxation of the hands as they move over the area exert a pumping action on the underlying capillaries and veins. This speeds up the flow of blood through the vessels so that waste products are removed and fresh blood delivers nutrients and oxygen more quickly. This will improve the condition of the tissues.

2 The flow of lymph through the lymph vessels and towards lymph nodes is speeded up in the same way. Thus, large particles of waste and tissue fluid are removed more quickly. This will reduce or prevent oedema.

3 Deep kneading has an effect on muscle tissue. The blood supply to muscles is improved. Waste products of fatigue are removed more quickly which will reduce pain and stiffness, particularly following exercise or sport. Fresh blood brings nutrients and oxygen to nourish muscle cells. This improves the tone and condition of the muscles and aids recovery. Slow, deep, rhythmic kneading will increase the blood supply and raise the temperature of the muscle, giving a feeling of warmth which eases tension and promotes relaxation. If the massage is performed deeply and vigorously, the muscles are warmed and stimulated. Warm muscles contract more efficiently and are more elastic than cold muscles – they are therefore less likely to suffer injury. Vigorous massage may therefore be used prior to sport or athletic activities to enhance performance and prevent injury. It should be used in conjunction with, but not instead of, warm-up and stretch routines.

4 Kneading mobilises tissues, increasing their extensibility and flexibility. It loosens tight fascia and adhesions, allowing free movement of muscle bundles.

5 Deep kneading will press the tissues against the bone. This will stimulate the blood supply to the periosteum and the bone, resulting in an increase in delivery of nutrients to the bone.

6 Palmar kneading also affects the condition of the

skin in a similar way to effleurage, i.e. the circulation to the skin is increased, producing hyperaemia and erythema. Therefore the condition and colour of the skin improves.

7 Sebaceous glands are stimulated to produce more sebum, which keeps the skin soft and supple.

8 The oil or cream used nourishes the skin.

9 The friction of the hands on the part and stimulation of mitosis increases the rate at which the cells of the stratum corneum are shed, which also improves the smoothness and condition of the skin.

10 Sweat glands are stimulated and excrete more sweat.

11 Kneading over the abdomen in the direction of movement of the contents of the colon will stimulate peristalsis.

USES

Palmar kneading is used:

1 to stimulate a sluggish circulation and prevent varicose veins and varicose ulcers

2 to stimulate lymphatic drainage and prevent or relieve oedema

3 to improve the condition of muscle tissue and maintain tone and elasticity

4 to warm up muscles prior to exercise, sport or athletic performance (warm-up and stretch exercise must follow)

5 to remove waste products of fatigue following exercise, sport or athletic performance, thus relieving stiffness and pain and promoting fast recovery

6 to promote muscle relaxation

7 to produce a sedative and general relaxing effect

8 to mobilise tissues and improve extensibility, loosen tight fascia and adhesions

9 to improve the condition of the skin

10 to increase alertness and feelings of well-being and prevent lethargy, if the movements are performed briskly

11 · to stimulate peristalsis and prevent or relieve constipation by kneading the abdomen in the direction of movement in the colon

DIGITAL AND THUMB KNEADING

Small circular movements are performed over small areas or small muscles using the pad of the thumb or the pads on the palmar surface of the first, second and third fingers. Again, the pressure must be applied in an upward direction, on half the circle, and then eased as the fingers come round and down. These digital movements are useful over the upper and middle fibres of the trapezius muscle, over the flexors and extensors of the forearm, down the erector spinae, around the colon, and over the pectoral muscles. Thumb movements are useful around the patella, over the anterior tibials, over the dorsum and sole of the foot, over the palmar and dorsal surface of the hand, and around the sacrum.

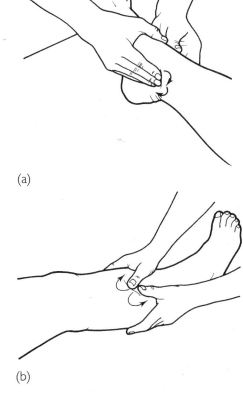

(a)

(b)

Figure 6.3 (a) digital kneading (b) thumb kneading

TECHNIQUE

◆ Select use of thumbs or digits depending on the area to be treated. Over smaller or confined areas such as the upper and middle fibres of trapezius, the thumbs are suitable but over larger areas such as over the length of erector spinae on either side of the spine, the digits are more suitable.

◆ Place the thumbs or the digits on the area.

◆ Select the depth of pressure according to the condition of the tissues and the type of massage.

◆ Perform small circular movements with the pressure on the upward part of the circle. Ease the pressure on the downward part but maintain contact.

◆ Do not hyper-extend the thumbs or fingers as the joints will be strained.

◆ Avoid repeating the pressure over the same area as

this may be painful for the client. Perform one circle and move smoothly and continuously to the adjoining area.

ULNAR BORDER KNEADING

This is similar in technique, effects and uses to digital kneading but the ulnar border of the hand is used to obtain greater depth. The ulnar border of the hand is placed on the part and moved in circles. It is used mainly over the soles of the feet and around the colon in abdominal massage. When performed around the colon the pressure changes; the pressure is upwards over the ascending colon (on the right side); the pressure is across over the transverse colon; and downwards over the descending colon (on the left side).

EFFECTS

1 The small kneading movements will increase the circulation to small localised areas, thus improving the condition of tissue.

2 They will mobilise localised areas and loosen adhesions.

3 Slow, rhythmical movements will promote relaxation and relieve pain over areas of tension and tension nodules.

4 They will increase lymphatic drainage in sluggish areas such as around the ankles.

USES

Digital, thumb and ulnar border kneading are used:

1 to stimulate circulation to small areas as explained above

2 to relieve pain and tension, especially over the trapezius and sacrum

3 to reduce fatigue and pain in the feet following prolonged standing

4 to break down or loosen adhesions.

Wringing

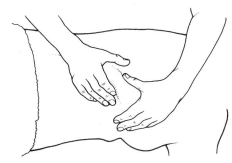

Figure 6.4 Wringing to the lateral aspect of the back

Wringing is a manipulation where the tissues are lifted away from the bone, and pushed and wrung from side to side as the hands move up and down. It must not be used on over-stretched muscles or those with poor tone.

TECHNIQUE

1 The stance is usually stride standing.

2 The hands must be warm, relaxed and supple.

3 The tissues are grasped in the palm of the hand and held between the fingers and thumb (taking care not to pinch).

4 The tissues are lifted away from the bone.

5 The tissues are moved diagonally from side to side by pushing the fingers of one hand towards the thumb of the opposite hand.

6 Keeping the tissues in the palm and lifted away from the bone, the hands move up and down along the length of the part, pushing the flesh from side to side. Do not pinch with the thumbs and fingers of the same hand.

7 The hands work up and down until the area is well covered and return to starting point.

Remember the fingers of the right hand work with the thumb of the left hand to press the flesh diagonally, then the fingers of the left hand move towards the thumb of the right hand. Wringing can only be performed over areas of loose or supple tissue which can be lifted away from the bone. Where tissues are firmly adhered to the bone, such as over the ribs or lateral aspect of the thigh where the fascia lata firmly binds the tissues, then wringing is difficult, ineffective and should be avoided.

EFFECTS

1 The alternate squeezing and releasing action of the hands on the tissues again increases the circulation to the area, removing waste products and bringing oxygen and nutrients to the area, thus improving the condition of the tissues.

2 Tissue fluid is squeezed from tissue spaces and the flow of lymph is speeded up.

3 The increased blood flow will increase metabolism and stimulate and improve the condition of the tissues.

4 The increased blood flow will raise the temperature of the area slightly, which will aid relaxation and relieve pain.

5 This manipulation improves the elasticity and extensibility of the tissues; it stretches tight fascia and tight muscle fibres. It is very useful for easing tension and mobilising large muscle groups, especially before and after exercise.

6 When used over areas of adipose tissue, it stimulates and helps to soften the area.

7 It has a sedative effect on nerve endings when performed in a slow, rhythmical relaxing manner, but it stimulates the area when performed briskly and vigorously.

USES

Wringing is used:

1 in conjunction with other manipulations to improve circulation and lymphatic flow

2 to warm tissues to ease tension and relieve pain

3 to improve the elasticity of skin and muscles

4 to stimulate, warm and soften areas of adipose tissue

5 to mobilise one tissue over another

6 to promote relaxation if performed slowly and rhythmically

7 to stimulate and invigorate if performed briskly.

Picking up

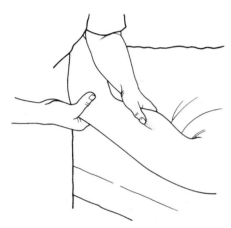

Figure 6.5 Single-handed picking up of biceps

Picking up is also a manipulation where the tissues are lifted away from the bone, squeezed and released. It may be performed with one hand or with both hands. It must not be used on stretched muscles or those with poor tone.

SINGLE-HANDED PICKING UP: TECHNIQUE

This method is performed with one hand grasping the muscle.

1 The stance is walk standing.

2 Spread the thumb away from the fingers, i.e. abduct the thumb.

3 Place the thumb on one side of the muscle or group and the fingers together on the other side.

4 Grasp and lift the muscle in the palm of the hand, squeezing with the thumb and fingers (do not pinch).

5 Release the muscle and move the hand forward, pushing upward with the palm and web of the abducted thumb. Slight flexion and extension of the wrist accompanies this movement.

6 The hand moves upwards in this manner, picking up, squeezing, releasing and moving on.

7 The hand may work up and down, or it may work up and slide back down.

8 Use the other hand to support the tissues.

REINFORCED PICKING UP: TECHNIQUE

For this method one hand is placed on the area as in single-handed work, but the other hand is placed over it to reinforce and provide more depth to the movement.

1 Place one hand (right if you are right handed) on the part, as explained in single-handed picking up.

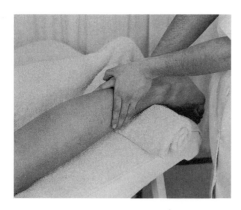

Figure 6.6 Reinforced picking up of gastrocnemius

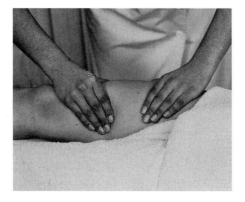

Figure 6.7 Double-handed picking up of thigh

2 Place the other hand over the top, with the thumb over the index finger of the underneath hand.

3 The hands then work together (like the wings of a bird) with the fingers of the right and left hand lifting, squeezing and releasing.

4 The elbows need to be fairly straight for this manipulation, as body weight is applied through the arms.

DOUBLE-HANDED PICKING UP:

TECHNIQUE

This is performed by two hands working in a synchronised manner up and down, usually on the large muscle groups of the leg or on adipose tissue at the sides of the trunk and hips.

1 The hands are placed on the area with the web of each abducted thumb facing towards each other, with the thumbs and fingers placed around the part and elbows out (abducted).

2 One hand starts lifting and squeezing the tissues (as before). On release of the tissues by this hand, the other performs the same action slightly above, maintaining the rhythm.

3 In this way the hands move up over the area in synchronised chugging movements.

4 The pressure upwards is emphasised by the hand which is pointing and working upwards in the direction of venous return.

EFFECTS AND USES

The effects and uses of picking up are as for wringing.

Skin rolling

This manipulation presses and rolls the skin and subcutaneous tissues against underlying bone.

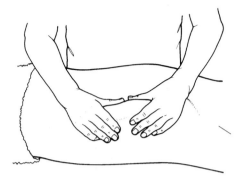

Figure 6.8 Skin rolling over ribs

Therefore it can only be performed where there is a bony framework underneath to work against. It is particularly effective when used transversely across the back, over the ribs or across the limbs.

TECHNIQUE

1 The stance is stride standing.

2 Place the hands flat over the area with the thumbs abducted.

3 Lift and push the flesh with the fingers towards the thumbs.

4 Roll this flesh, using the thumbs moving across towards the fingers.

5 Move smoothly onto a lower area and then work back.

EFFECTS

These are mainly on the skin and subcutaneous tissue.

1 Skin rolling increases blood flow to the skin, thus producing an erythema.

2 The increased blood flow delivers nutrients and oxygen to the skin cells and removes waste products more quickly, thus improving the condition of the skin.

3 The oil or cream used nourishes the skin and improves its suppleness.

4 As the skin is moved over underlying tissues, its elasticity and suppleness is improved. This will help to soften established scar tissue.

5 The friction of the hands on the part aids desquamation.

6 Skin rolling stimulates and softens areas of subcutaneous fat.

7 It stimulates sebaceous glands to produce more sebum.

8 It stimulates sweat glands to excrete more sweat.

USES

Skin rolling is used:

1 to improve the condition of the skin

2 to improve suppleness and elasticity of the skin

3 to soften and stimulate areas of subcutaneous fat

4 to soften and mobilise scar tissue

5 to induce relaxation if performed slowly

6 to stimulate and invigorate if performed briskly.

Muscle rolling

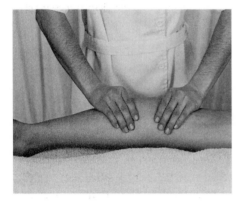

Figure 6.9 Muscle rolling on calf

This manipulation lifts the muscle away from the bone and moves it from side to side in a rocking manner.

TECHNIQUE

1 The stance is stride standing.

2 Place the thumbs nail to nail in a straight line on one side of the muscle and place the fingers over the other side.

3 Grasp and lift the muscle away from the bone.

4 Push the muscle with the thumbs towards the fingers, which give slightly as the muscle moves.

5 Push the muscle back towards the thumbs, using the fingers in the same way.

6 Push the muscle backwards and forwards, applying pressure into the muscle and using a rocking action.

7 Move along the muscle by sliding the hands.

EFFECTS

1 Muscle rolling stimulates the circulation if performed briskly.

2 It improves lymphatic flow and drainage of tissue fluid.

3 It improves elasticity and extensibility in the muscle.

4 It releases tension in muscle fibres when performed slowly and rhythmically. It is particularly useful if pain is present in a muscle. Gentle muscle rolling can be tolerated and will ease the pain, allowing other movements such as effleurage or gentle kneading to be performed.

USES

Muscle rolling is used:

1 to warm muscles and improve elasticity prior to sporting or athletic performance

2 to relieve pain and stiffness in muscles, particularly following sporting and athletic performance. This manipulation is particularly useful when muscles are very painful and sore and unable to tolerate any other pressure manipulations. The muscle is carefully grasped and very gently and rhythmically rocked to and fro until pain and tension are eased.

Frictions

These are very localised manipulations performed with the fingers or thumb. They may be applied transversely across muscle fibres or in a circular movement. They are deep movements performed with much pressure. The pressure may be selected at the commencement and kept constant throughout, as is usual with transverse frictions, or the pressure may get progressively deeper, as with circular frictions. The pressure must, however, be completely released before moving on to a new area. Frictions are performed on dry skin, free of oil or talcum powder, so that the fingers move the skin and do not slip over it.

Remember these are specialised movements, used when localised depth and pressure is required. They should not be confused with digital or thumb kneading, which apply constant upward pressure using a circular movement.

Fast stroking is also sometimes referred to as brisk friction because the hands do apply friction to the area, but this covers a large area and is not localised.

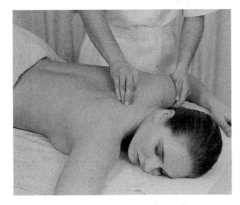

Figure 6.10 Circular frictions to tension nodules in trapezius

Circular frictions: technique

These are small circular movements performed by the fingers or thumb.

1 The stance is usually walk standing.

2 Select and examine the small localised area where frictions are required.

3 Stroke it gently with the sweeping thumb or palm.

4 Use the thumb or the fingers; the middle finger is usually used to reinforce the index and ring fingers.

5 Do not hyper-extend any joints when applying pressure, as this will strain and damage the joints. Keep the fingers straight.

6 Circular frictions are performed in small circles, moving deeper and deeper into the tissues to a maximum depth, then release. Repeat three to four times over the same spot and then move to another area as required.

7 The fingers or thumb must not slide or rub over the surface of the skin, but the superficial tissues must move with the fingers over the deeper ones.

8 Areas requiring frictions may be tender and care must be taken not to cause unnecessary pain through excessive pressure.

9 Effleurage or stroke the area frequently between friction manipulations and at the end of the treatment.

Transverse frictions: technique

These are backward and forward transverse movements performed across ligaments or joints.

1 The stance is stride standing or walk standing.

2 Select the area requiring frictions.

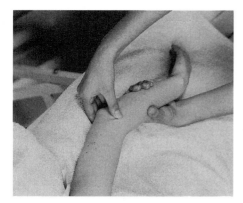

Figure 6.11 Transverse frictions to the extensor tendon

3 Use the thumb or fingers as before.

4 Take care not to hyper-extend the joints, particularly those of the thumb – this is so easily done when pressure is applied.

5 For transverse frictions, the pressure is selected at the commencement and is maintained throughout the movements – it does not get deeper.

6 Place the thumb or fingers at right angles to the part, e.g. the ligament or muscle fibres, and move transversely across it, forwards and backwards six to eight times. Release and repeat.

7 Take care not to cause unnecessary pain by selecting too deep a pressure.

8 Effleurage or stroke the area frequently.

EFFECTS

1 Friction increases the circulation to localised areas, producing an erythema.

2 When friction is performed over ligaments and around joints the circulation to the area is increased, improving nourishment of ligaments and joint structure, and improving their function.

3 Movement of the tissues over one another will break down adhesions and mobilise fibrous tissue.

4 Deep frictions will break down and disperse fibrous nodules and ease fibrositic conditions.

5 Friction massage will improve the extensibility of old scar tissue and help to free scars from underlying tissues.

6 When performed on either side of the spine it will stimulate spinal nerves, producing feelings of invigoration.

USES

Friction is used:

1 to increase local circulation and promote healing

2 around joints to loosen adhesions and improve movement

3 to stretch and loosen old scar tissue

4 to disperse tension nodules, found particularly in the upper and middle fibres of the trapezius

5 to increase the circulation and promote healing of chronic tendon strains, such as tennis or golfer's elbow

6 to stimulate and invigorate lethargic clients when performed along each side of the spine.

?

1 Name the five manipulations that belong to the petrissage group.

2 Explain what is meant by the following:
   (a) digital kneading
   (b) thumb kneading
   (c) ulnar border kneading.

3 List four types of palmar kneading.

4 Describe the effects of palmar kneading.

5 Give six uses of kneading.

6 State briefly how the tissues are manipulated in wringing.

7 Explain briefly why the temperature of the area is slightly raised when massaged.

8 Give six effects of wringing.

9 List six uses of wringing.

10 Explain briefly the difference between reinforced picking up and double-handed picking up.

11 Give the main tissue affected by skin rolling.

12 List six uses of skin rolling.

13 Explain the technique of muscle rolling.

14 Give one condition where muscle rolling is particularly effective.

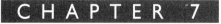

CHAPTER 7

Percussion and vibration groups

• •

OBJECTIVES

After you have studied this chapter you will be able to:

1 list the four manipulations of the percussion group
2 describe the technique for each manipulation
3 explain the effects of each manipulation
4 explain the uses of each manipulation
5 identify areas of the body where the manipulation would be effective
6 state conditions or areas of the body where these manipulations should not be used
7 perform each manipulation on appropriate areas of the body
8 state the difference between vibration and shaking
9 describe the techniques of vibration and shaking
10 list the effects and uses of vibration and shaking.

Percussion (tapotement) group

As their name suggests, all the manipulations of this group strike or tap the part. The hands are used alternately to strike the tissues with light, springy, rhythmical movements. When performing these manipulations, particular care must be taken to avoid bony prominences, ridges or areas where the bone is not well covered. They must not be performed on old or very thin clients, or those with loose, poorly toned muscles and little adipose tissue.

These manipulations are never used in a relaxing massage because they are too vigorous and stimulating.

There are four manipulations in this group, named

according to the position of the hands and the way in which they strike the part:

1 hacking

2 cupping

3 beating

4 pounding.

Hacking

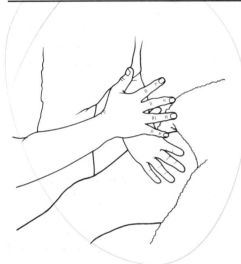

Figure 7.1 Hacking

This manipulation uses the ulnar border of the hand and the little finger, ring and middle fingers to strike the tissues in a light, springy, brisk manner. The forearm must alternately pronate and supinate to allow the fingers to strike the part. The hands strike alternately.

It is important to avoid flexion and extension of the elbow joint as the resulting 'chopping' action is too heavy and powerful. This is a difficult manipulation to master and much practice is needed to perfect it. It can be practised initially on a pillow and the technique perfected before performing on a client. There are certain procedures to practise which will lead to correct and skilful technique.

TECHNIQUE

1 The stance should be stride standing, with the feet a good distance apart and the knees relaxed or bent, keeping the back straight.

2 Place the hands together with the fingers straight as in prayer, thumbs against chest.

3 Take the elbows away from the sides, i.e. abduct the shoulder joint. The wrists will now be extended at an 80–90° angle.

4 Place the arms parallel and just above the part to be worked on.

5 Supinate and pronate the forearm so that the little fingers strike the part lightly and then lift away.

6 Practise this action until the arms roll easily.

7 Now practise the whole procedure. Part the hands and strike the part alternately (remember to keep the elbows out and wrists extended).

8 Relax or slightly flex the fingers and, keeping the same action, strike the part alternately with the ulnar border of the little, ring and middle fingers.

9 Strike lightly, briskly and rhythmically with alternate hands.

10 Work up and down or across an area – cover thoroughly.

11 The hands may also diverge – the heels of the hand stay close but the fingers diverge forming a '\ /' shape. This is useful over the upper fibres of the trapezius, below the nape of the neck.

EFFECTS

The effects are similar for all the percussion manipulations, except that beating and pounding are heavier manipulations and produce deeper effects.

1 Hacking increases the circulation to the area, producing hyperaemia (increase in blood flow) and erythema (reddening of the skin).

2 It stimulates and softens areas of adipose tissue and is very effective on areas of hard fat and cellulite.

3 Hacking stimulates reflex contraction of muscle fibres and may increase muscle tone. It must be performed lightly and briskly. Because the other manipulations are not as brisk and sharp, they do not produce as great an effect.

4 The increased blood flow warms the area and increases the metabolic rate.

5 Hacking down either side of the spine stimulates spinal nerves and is generally invigorating.

USES

Hacking is used:

1 to increase circulation to the area

2 to warm an area

3 to stimulate and soften areas of fat

4 to invigorate and give a feeling of glow and well-being

5 to stimulate muscles with poor tone.

Cupping

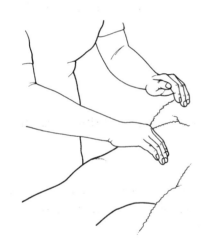

Figure 7.2 Cupping

Cupping (also known as clapping) is performed using the cupped hands to strike the part alternately. The movements are light and brisk, producing a hollow sound.

Technique

1 The stance is stride standing, as for hacking.

2 Make a hollow shape with the hand by flexing the metacarpo-phalangeal joints (knuckle joints). Keep the thumb in contact with the index finger.

3 Straighten the elbows – they may flex and extend slightly with the movement.

4 Place the hands on the part.

5 Flex and extend the wrist as the hands lift up and down alternately; keep the wrists loose and flexible.

6 Strike the part lightly and briskly with the fingers, part of the palm and heel of the hand.

7 The hands should clap the area, making a hollow sound. Avoid a slapping noise which will occur if the hands are too flat. This will sting and be uncomfortable for the client.

8 Work up and down or across the area. Cover it thoroughly four to six times until an erythema is produced.

Effects and uses

The effects and uses of cupping are similar to those of hacking, but cupping is not as effective for stimulating muscle contraction.

Beating

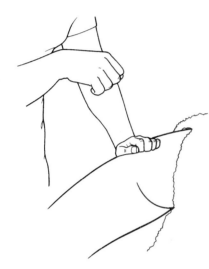

Figure 7.3 Beating

This is a heavier percussion movement which is useful on very large heavy areas of adipose tissue, particularly over the buttocks and thighs. The manipulation is performed by striking the area with a loosely clenched fist. The back of the fingers and heel of the hands strike the part as the hands alternately drop heavily onto the area.

Technique

1. The stance is stride standing.

2. Loosely clench the fingers: keep the thumb against the hand.

3. Straighten the elbows.

4. Place the loosely clenched hands on the part so that the back of the fingers and heel of the hand lie in contact with the part.

5. Extend and flex the wrist and lift the arms slightly so that the hands fall alternately and heavily on the part.

6. Work up and down or across the area and ensure that you cover it thoroughly four to six times.

7. The movement should be brisk and rhythmical. The pressure can vary from light to heavy, depending on the required outcome and the type of tissue being worked on. Well-toned bulky muscles or a depth of adipose tissue (fat) will be suitable for heavier pressure.

8. It is usual to work with both hands striking the part alternately, but it is possible over small or awkward areas to use one hand only, supporting the tissues with the other.

EFFECTS AND USES

These are similar to hacking, but beating is heavier and is particularly effective in stimulating and softening adipose tissue.

Pounding

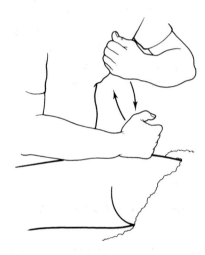

Figure 7.4 Pounding

This, again, is a heavy percussion movement, performed by the ulnar border (little finger side) of the loosely clenched fist. The side of the hands strike the part alternately.

TECHNIQUE

1. The stance is stride standing.
2. Loosely clench the fingers.
3. Place the ulnar border of the hands on the part, with one hand slightly in front of the other.
4. Lift the front hand and strike behind the back hand as the back hand lifts off the part.
5. Continue to circle the hands over each other, striking the part alternately with each hand.
6. The movement should be brisk and rhythmical. The pressure can vary from light to heavy, depending on the desired effect and density of tissue.
7. Cover the area thoroughly four to six times, or until the desired erythema reaction is achieved.

EFFECTS AND USES

The effects and uses of pounding are as for beating, cupping and hacking.

Vibration group

There are two manipulations in this group: shaking and vibration. Both produce vibrations or tremors within the tissues. Shaking is a much bigger, coarser movement and produces shaking of the muscle, while vibrations are fine movements which merely produce a tremor.

Shaking

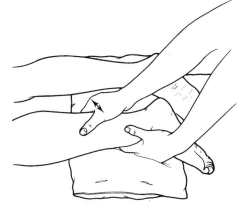

Figure 7.5 Shaking

This manipulation may be performed with one hand grasping and shaking the muscle while the other supports the part. It may also be performed with both hands working together, pushing in and out in a shaking action. This is particularly effective performed over the chest to loosen secretions and mucous in the lungs.

Technique

1 The stance is walk standing.

2 Support the part with the other hand so that the muscle is relaxed.

3 Grasp the muscle, usually towards its distal end. Lift it between the thumb and fingers, being careful not to pinch.

4 Shake the muscle gently from side to side. As the muscle relaxes, a greater degree of movement will be possible.

Effect

Gentle shaking will aid muscle relaxation, which will reduce pain and stiffness.

Uses

Shaking is used to relieve pain and stiffness in muscles, particularly after exercise or athletic performance.

Note: shaking of the chest to loosen secretions requires the correct positioning for drainage of lung secretions and is not covered in this book.

Vibration

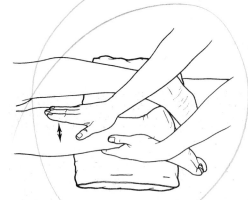

Figure 7.6 Vibration

This manipulation is usually performed with one hand. However, on large areas both hands can be used. The hand is placed over the area and vibrated either up and down or from side to side. The action produces vibrations in the underlying tissue.

TECHNIQUE

1 The stance is walk standing or stride standing.

2 Support the part with one hand.

3 Place the other hand on the part.

4 Keep the fingers straight and the thumb adducted.

5 Vibrate the hand up and down or from side to side to produce a tremor in the tissues. The hand maintains contact throughout.

6 Avoid tension developing in the working hand, arm and shoulder.

7 The vibrations may be static and performed in one area only, or they may run or move over the part.

8 On small areas, and when very fine tremors are required, the finger tips only can be used to vibrate up and down or from side to side.

EFFECTS

1 Vibration aids absorption of tissue fluid.

2 It soothes superficial nerves, which relieves tension and promotes relaxation.

3 When performed along the colon, it will relieve flatulence.

USES

Vibration is used:

1 to stimulate sluggish lymphatic drainage

2 to relieve tension and aid relaxation

3 to relieve flatulence.

?

1 List the manipulations in the percussion group.

2 Name conditions when percussion manipulations would not be suitable.

3 Describe the technique of hacking.

4 Explain the effects of the percussion group.

5 Give four uses of this group.

6 Give one condition where beating and pounding are particularly effective.

7 Explain the effects of shaking and vibration on the tissues.

8 Give three uses of vibration movements.

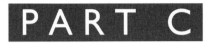

PART C

Massage routines and adaptations

....

CHAPTER 8

Massage routines

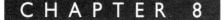

After you have studied this chapter you will be able to:

1 give the approximate timing for each area when giving a general body massage
2 visualise the tissues in the areas being massaged
3 identify the principal lymph nodes
4 discuss the importance of continuity, depth, speed and rhythm and how they should be varied
5 select an appropriate form of massage to suit different conditions
6 perform a variety of manipulations on all areas of the body.

Basic guidelines

The timing of a body massage is usually one hour but may be longer. The order of covering the body is usually:

right leg	7 minutes
left leg	7 minutes
left arm	5 minutes
right arm	5 minutes
décolleté	5 minutes
abdomen	5 minutes
back of legs	6 minutes
back	20 minutes

These timings are approximate and will vary to suit client needs. More attention may be required on some areas than others. For example, if there was oedema of the ankles then a longer time would be spent on the legs.

When performing massage it is important to mentally visualise the tissues that the hands are moving over and to sense variations in tension or abnormal structure through the hands. A knowledge of the anatomical structure of the area is therefore essential. The following text identifies the important structures, lists suggested massage routines and highlights areas where special care is needed. The lists of manipulations are suggestions only. Manipulations should be selected to suit the client and personal preference or expertise. There are, however, basic rules and guidelines.

1 **Comfort**: massage must always be comfortable. It must not hurt or injure the client, even the vigorous and stimulating techniques.

2 **Direction**: pressure must be applied in the direction of venous drainage towards the heart and the direction of lymphatic drainage to the nearest lymph nodes. (Do not pull back what you have pushed along as this is counter-productive.)

3 **Order**: begin with effleurage, follow with applicable petrissage manipulations then percussion if suitable, and complete with effleurage. Effleurage and stroking may be interspersed with any of the manipulations.

4 **Continuity**: massage should be continuous – the transition between strokes should be barely perceptible. The hands should not be lifted off the area once treatment has commenced until that area is completed. Move smoothly from one stroke to another.

5 **Speed**: this must be selected according to the type of massage required – slow for relaxing, moderate for a general massage, and faster for a vigorous, stimulating massage.

6 **Depth**: this must be selected according to the type of massage, as above – moderate depth for a relaxing and general massage, deeper for a vigorous massage. Depth must also be adjusted to suit the client and the desired outcome of the treatment. For example, young, fit clients will take greater depth than older clients; well-toned clients will take greater depth than those with loose, flabby muscles or thin clients; obese clients or those with specific areas of hard adipose tissue will require greater depth. Those accustomed to massage generally prefer a deeper massage than new nervous clients. (Always ask the client if manipulations are too deep or not deep enough.)

7 **Rhythm**: this must be consistent regardless of the type of client. The rhythm is selected at the beginning of the massage and maintained throughout, e.g. slow rhythm for a relaxing massage, moderate for a general, and a faster rhythm for a vigorous massage.

8 **Stance**: protect yourself from strain and injury by adopting the correct posture. There are two standing positions used in massage:

(a) walk standing (i.e. with one foot in front of the other) is used when massaging up and down the length of the body

(b) stride standing (i.e. with the feet apart) is used when working across the body.

Always keep the back straight and the shoulders relaxed. Allow the knees to bend when necessary to apply body weight and to reach all areas. Increased depth and pressure must come from body weight transmitted through the arms, but not by pushing with the arms. Use a slight swaying body movement to achieve this. Keep the feet apart – this improves balance and provides stability, as it gives a wider base.

9 **Concentration**: maintain your concentration throughout the massage. Although massage movements become semi-automatic as expertise develops, it is still important to concentrate fully on the task in hand. Continuity and rhythm will suffer if there is a lapse in concentration, and this is transmitted to the client.

10 **Coverage**: cover the whole area thoroughly. Do not neglect small areas as this will result in uneven coverage.

Practise all massage manipulations at various speeds, depths and rhythms. Practise on fellow therapists until you have perfected the technique. Ask the model to comment on or criticise your performance. Change over roles and work with different people – this will enable you to sense and feel the differences in technique and judge the most effective. Practise on different types of flesh – well toned and poorly toned, young and old, thin and obese, etc.

Leg

BONES

The leg contains the following bones:

◆ **femur**: thigh bone

◆ **tibia**: medial and larger bone of the lower leg

◆ **fibula**: lateral and thinner bone of the lower leg

◆ **patella**: small bone on front of the knee joint which

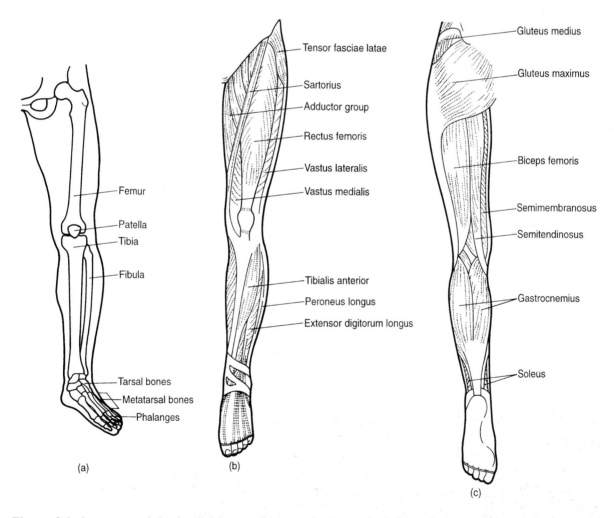

Figure 8.1 Anatomy of the leg (a) bones (b) muscles (anterior) (c) muscles (posterior)

allows the patella tendon of the quadriceps muscle to move smoothly over the knee joint

◆ **tarsals**, **metatarsals** and **phalanges** of the ankle and foot.

JOINTS

Table 8.1 Classification of leg joints

Name	Type	Movement
Hip	Ball-and-socket (synovial), formed by acetabulum of innominate bone and the head of the femur	Flexion, extension, abduction, adduction, rotation (medial and lateral) and circumduction
Knee	Hinge (synovial), formed by the condyles of the femur and the condyles of the tibia	Flexion and extension
Ankle	Hinge (synovial), lower end of tibia and fibula and talus	Dorsi flexion (foot up) and plantar flexion (point foot)
Intertarsal	Gliding (synovial) between tarsal bones	Inversion (turn foot in) and eversion (turn foot out)
Metatarso-phalangeal	Condyloid (synovial)	Flexion, extension, abduction, adduction and circumduction
Inter-phalangeal of toes	Hinge (synovial)	Flexion and extension

MUSCLES

Table 8.2 Classification of leg muscles

Name	Position	Action
Thigh		
Sartorius	Diagonally across front of thigh	Flexes the hip and knee joint
Quadriceps group (4)	Front of thigh	Large powerful group which extend the knee joint and keep it straight when weight bearing
Rectus femoris	Front of thigh (superficial)	
Vastus medialis	Medial aspect of thigh	
Vastus lateralis	Lateral aspect of thigh	
Vastus intermedius	Front of thigh, deep	

Table 8.2 continued

Name	Position	Action

Hamstrings (3)
  Biceps femoris
  Semimembranosus
  Semitendinosus
	Back of thigh	Work as a group to extend the hip joint and flex the knee joint

Adductors (5)
  Adductor magnus
  Adductor longus
  Adductor brevis
  Pectineus
  Gracilis
	Medial aspect of thigh	Work as a group to adduct the hip joint (pull inwards) and rotate it laterally

Abductors (3)
  Gluteus medius
  Gluteus minimus
	Outer buttock region	Work as a group to abduct the hip joint and rotate it medially.

Tensor fascia lata	Upper outer thigh	(Tensor fascia lata also tenses the band of fascia on the lateral apsect of the thigh)
Gluteus maximus	Large superficial buttock muscle	Extends the hip joint

Lower leg

Name	Position	Action

Anterior tibials (3)
  Tibialis anterior
  Extensor hallucis longus
  Extensor digitorum longus
	Antero-lateral aspect of lower leg	All dorsi flex the foot and invert it. Extensor hallucis longus extends the big toe. Extensor digitorum extends other toes

Posterior tibials (5) Gastrocnemius	Superficial calf muscle	Flexes the knee joint; plantar flexes the foot
Soleus	Deep to gastrocnemius and in the calf	Plantar flexes the foot
Tibialis posterior Flexor hallucis longus	Deep muscles of the calf	Plantar flexes the foot Flexor hallucis longus flexes the big toe
Flexor digitorum longus		Flexor digitorum flexes the other toes

Peronei (3)
  Peroneus longus
  Peroneus brevis
  Peroneus tertious
	Lateral aspect of lower leg	Dorsi flex the foot and evert it

Numerous small muscles lie in layers in the sole of the foot and between the metatarsals.

LYMPHATIC DRAINAGE

There are two groups of nodes in the leg:

- **popliteal nodes**: behind the knee, into which the lymph from the lower leg drains
- **inguinal nodes**: in the groin, into which lymph from the leg drains.

BLOOD SUPPLY

Main arteries
Blood is carried to the leg by the large femoral artery and its branches.

Main veins
Blood is carried from the legs by the great and small saphenous veins, the femoral vein and its branches.

POINTS TO CONSIDER

- On the anterior surface of the lower leg the anterior border of the tibia, commonly known as the shin, is protected only by skin and fascia (fibrous tissue). It forms a bony ridge down the front of the lower leg and must be avoided during massage as pressure on the bone may cause pain and discomfort. The anterior tibial muscles lie on the lateral aspect of this bone (i.e. towards the outside) and any kneading movements should be concentrated over this outer leg area.

- The medial and lateral malleoli on either side of the ankle joint must also be avoided, as must the patella on the front of the knee. Massage movements should be performed around these bony points, avoiding direct pressure.

- On the anterior surface of the thigh the large bulky quadriceps muscle and the adductors on the medial aspect are suitable for any of the massage manipulations. However, the upper third of the medial aspect, known as the **femoral triangle**, is a very sensitive area and must be avoided.

◆ The lateral outer aspect of the thigh has a tight band of fascia, namely the fascia lata, passing from the muscle-tensor fascia lata down to the knee joint. This binds the tissues tightly, making it impossible to perform wringing, picking up or skin rolling on the outer thigh unless there is a depth of covering fat.

◆ The buttock and outer thigh area may be covered with adipose tissue (fat). In obese people the anterior and medial aspects of the thigh may also be covered. These areas can take the heavier manipulations of hacking, cupping, beating and pounding. Always ensure that you avoid the bony prominence of the greater trochanter on the outer aspect, just below and lateral to the groin.

MASSAGE ROUTINE

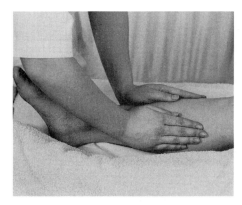

Figure 8.2 Efleurage to lower leg

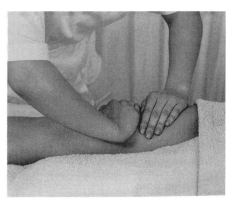

Figure 8.3 Deep effleurage to thigh

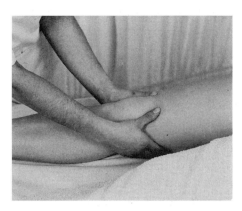

Figure 8.4 Thumb kneading around the patella

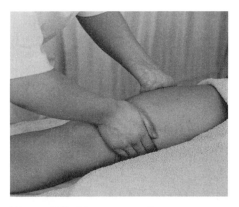

Figure 8.5 Alternate palmar kneading to abductors and adductors

The suggested massage routine for the leg is as follows:

- effleurage (front, sides and back)
- deeper effleurage over thigh
- alternate palmar kneading over abductors and adductors
- reinforced or double-handed kneading over quadriceps
- wringing to thigh (medial to lateral and back)
- picking up – reinforced or double handed
- deep effleurage to thigh
- thumb kneading around patella
- effleurage to lower leg
- thumb kneading to anterior tibials (lateral to shin bone)
- alternate palmar kneading to calf
- stroking to dorsal surface of foot
- digital kneading around malleoli
- thumb kneading between metatarsals
- kneading to toes
- ulnar border kneading to sole of foot
- thumb kneading to sole of foot
- effleurage to whole leg.

Hacking and cupping are added to the thigh for a more invigorating massage, but not for a relaxing one.

BACK OF LEG

This is performed after the abdomen, when the client has turned over, and before the back routine.

- effleurage to back of leg and buttock
- deep effleurage to thigh and buttock
- double-handed kneading to thigh and buttock
- reinforced kneading to top of thigh and buttock

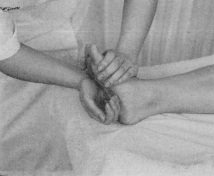

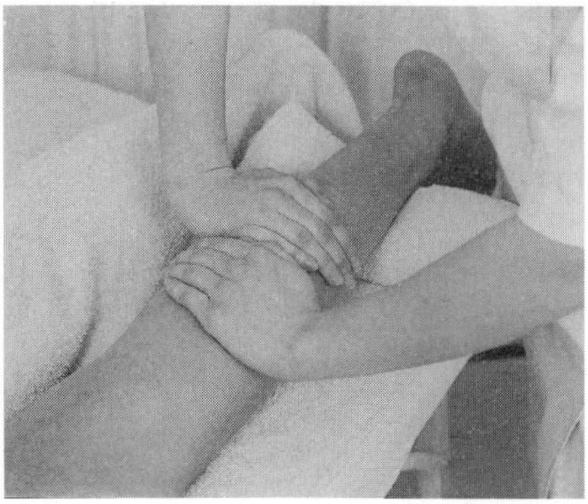

Figure 8.6 Ulnar border kneading to the sole

Figure 8.7 Effleurage of back of leg

- ◆ double-handed picking up to hamstrings
- ◆ deep effleurage to thigh and buttock
- ◆ effleurage to calf
- ◆ reinforced kneading to calf
- ◆ wringing to calf
- ◆ reinforced or single-handed picking up to calf
- ◆ effleurage to calf
- ◆ effleurage to leg.

Hacking, cupping, beating and pounding are used on the buttock for an invigorating massage and for treatment of cellulite.

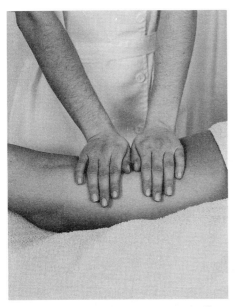

Figure 8.8 Double handed kneading to hamstrings

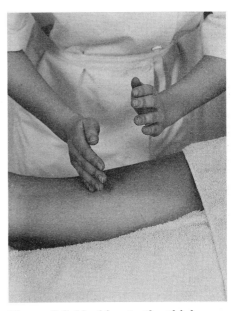

Figure 8.9 Hacking to the thigh

Arm

BONES

The arm contains the following bones:

- **humerus**: bone of the upper arm
- **radius**: lateral bone of the forearm
- **ulna**: medial bone of the forearm
- **carpals**, **metacarpals** and **phalanges** of the wrists and hands.

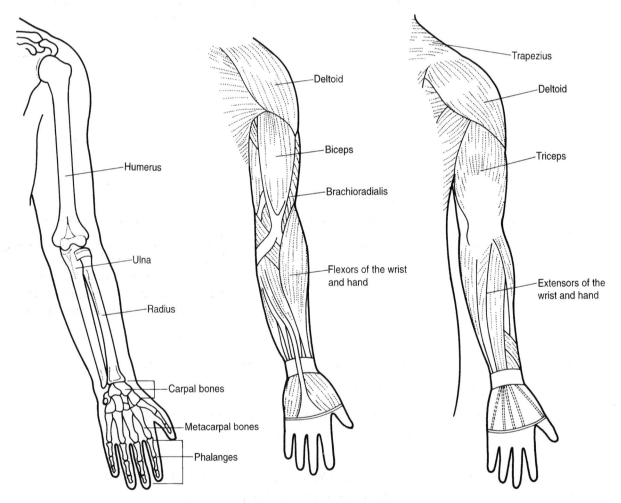

Figure 8.10 Anatomy of the arm (a) bones (b) muscles (anterior) (c) muscles (posterior)

JOINTS

Table 8.3 Classification of arm joints

Name	Type	Movement
Shoulder	Ball-and-socket (synovial), formed by the glenoid cavity of the scapula and the head of the humerus	Flexion, extension, abduction, adduction, rotation (medial and lateral) and circumduction
Elbow	Hinge (synovial)	Flexion and extension
Radio-ulnar joint	Pivot (synovial)	Pronation and supination
Wrist joint	Condyloid (synovial)	Flexion, extension, abduction, adduction and circumduction
Metacarpo-phalangeal	Condyloid (synovial)	Flexion, extension, abduction, adduction and circumduction
Interphalangeal	Hinge (synovial)	Flexion and extension

MUSCLES

Table 8.4 Classification of arm muscles

Name	Position	Action
Deltoid	Covers the shoulder	Three sets of fibres: anterior fibres flex shoulder joint; middle fibres abduct shoulder joint; posterior fibres extend shoulder joint
Triceps	Posterior aspect of upper arm	Extends elbow joint
Biceps	Anterior aspect of upper arm	Flexes elbow joint
Brachialis and brachioradialis	Deep to biceps	Flex elbow joint
Flexors of the wrist and fingers	Many muscles lie in layers on the anterior aspect of the forearm	Flex wrist and fingers
Extensors of the wrist and fingers	Many muscles lie in layers on the posterior aspect of the forearm	Extend wrist and fingers

Small muscles of the hand lie in the palm and also form the thenar eminence on the thumb side and the hypothenar eminence on the little finger side. Other small muscles lie between the metacarpals.

LYMPHATIC DRAINAGE

There are two groups of nodes in the arm:

◆ **supra trochlear**: at the elbow, drains the forearm

◆ **axillary**: in the axilla (armpit), drains lymph from arm.

BLOOD SUPPLY

Main arteries

Blood is carried to the arm by the axillary artery, the brachial artery, the radial artery and the ulnar artery.

Main veins

Blood is carried from the arm by the cephalic vein, the basilic vein, the brachial vein and the axillary vein.

POINTS TO CONSIDER

◆ Deltoid is a muscle made up of three sets of fibres: one on the front of the shoulder joint; one over the top; and one on the back of the joint. Therefore, kneading of this muscle must cover all these areas.

◆ There is very little tissue on the lateral aspect of the upper arm and deep massage can be painful. Make sure that you are actually working in the correct area for the biceps and triceps. The biceps is easily found on the anterior aspect of the upper arm. The triceps is more difficult to find as the arm rotates laterally. It lies on the posterior surface, so find the olecranon process (funny bone) and work directly above it.

◆ When kneading on the forearm, remember that the flexors originate at the medial epicondyle, so on the anterior surface begin your kneading towards the medial side and work slightly across and down. On the posterior surface the extensors originate from the lateral epicondyle, so begin kneading from the lateral side. Knead around the styloid processes at the wrist.

MASSAGE ROUTINE

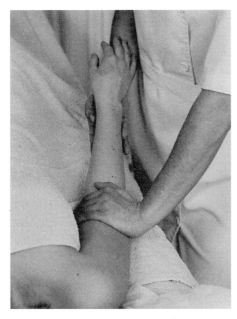

Figure 8.11 Effleurage of the arm

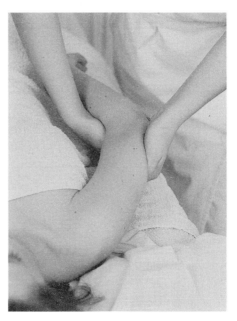

Figure 8.12 Single-handed kneading to triceps

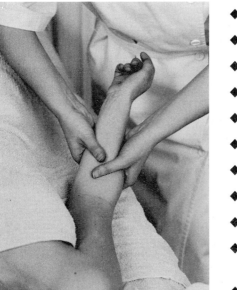

Figure 8.13 Thumb kneading to flexors of wrist and hand

The suggested massage routine for the arm is as follows:

♦ effleurage (front and back)

♦ alternate palmar kneading over deltoid

♦ single-handed kneading to triceps

♦ single-handed kneading to biceps

♦ wringing to triceps (if suitable)

♦ wringing to biceps (if suitable)

♦ stroking to upper arm (figure of eight)

♦ effleurage to forearm

♦ thumb kneading to flexors of wrist (anterior aspect)

♦ thumb kneading to extensors of wrist (posterior aspect)

♦ thumb kneading around styloid processes

♦ thumb kneading between metacarpals (dorsal aspect)

◆ kneading to fingers

◆ thumb kneading to thenar and hypothenar eminences and palm

◆ effleurage to arm.

Hacking may be performed on biceps and triceps for an invigorating massage.

Chest and abdomen

BONES

The chest contains the following bones:

◆ **sternum**: breast bone

◆ **clavicle**: collar bone

◆ **ribs**: 12 pairs.

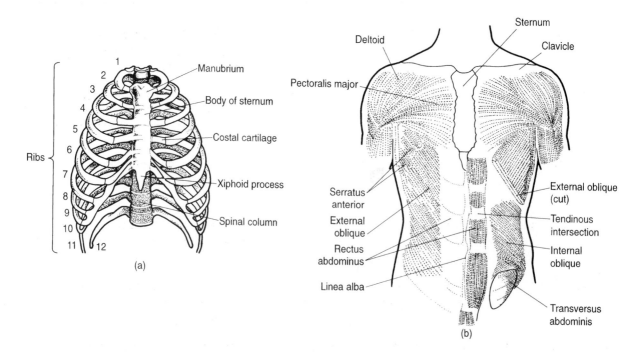

Figure 8.14 Anatomy of chest and abdomen (a) bones of thorax (b) muscles

JOINTS

Table 8.5 Classification of chest joints

Name	Type	Movement
Sterno-clavicular	Gliding (synovial) between the clavicle and sternum	Accompanies shoulder joint and girdle movements
Acromio-clavicular	Gliding (synovial) between the clavicle and acromion process of scapula	Accompanies shoulder joint and girdle movements

The ribs join the sternum via the costal cartilages and form a cage which protects the heart and lungs. There is no bony protection for the abdomen and its contents.

MUSCLES

Table 8.6 Classification of muscles of the chest and abdomen

Name	Position	Action
Chest		
Pectoralis major	Covers the chest	Flexes the shoulder joint and medially rotates it. Protracts the shoulder girdle
Pectoralis minor	Smaller and deep to pectoralis major	Holds the tip of the shoulder down during arm movements
Abdominal wall		
Rectus abdominis	Column of muscle, one on each side of midline	Flexes the trunk; one side working, side flexes the trunk
External oblique	Flat sheet of muscle passing obliquely down and in from ribs to pelvis and midline	Rotates the trunk to the opposite side; one side working aids side flexion of the trunk
Internal oblique	Flat sheet of muscle passing obliquely upwards and in from pelvis to midline and ribs	Rotates the trunk to the same side; one side working aids side flexion of the trunk
Transversus abdominis	Flat sheet of muscle passing transversely across the abdomen	Compresses the abdomen; used in all expulsive actions

Lymphatic drainage

There are three groups of nodes in the chest and abdomen:

◆ **axillary nodes**: in the axilla, into which lymph from the chest region drains

◆ **inguinal nodes**: in the groin

◆ **iliac nodes**: in the abdomen, into which lymph from the abdomen drains.

Blood supply

Main arteries
Blood is carried to the chest region via the subclavian artery and to the abdomen via the common iliac artery.

Main veins
Blood is carried from the chest via the superior vena cava. Blood is carried from the abdomen via the inferior vena cava.

Points to consider

◆ Avoid pressure over the clavicle; work below. The clavicular glands which lie in the décolleté above and below the clavicle may become very tender in the pre-menstrual female and pressure should be kept very light. Always ask the client if she feels tender or sore when touched and adapt the massage accordingly.

◆ The abdomen has no bony framework for protection and the underlying abdominal organs will be affected by the massage. If muscle tone of the abdominals is poor, or if they are loose and over-stretched, then manipulations and pressure must be light. If the muscles are well toned or covered by layers of adipose tissue (fat) then deeper pressure may be used. Heavy percussion movements should be avoided over the abdomen and chest.

◆ Massage will stimulate peristalsis (the movement of alternate contraction and relaxation of the intestines) and is frequently used to aid movement through the colon. Pressure must therefore be applied in the direction of movement through the colon. This pressure must be upwards on the right hand side of the abdomen over the ascending colon; from right to left along the transverse colon, just below the waist; and downwards on the left side along the descending colon. Make sure that the pressure is correct when kneading or stroking the colon.

MASSAGE ROUTINES

The following are suggested massage routines for the chest and abdomen.

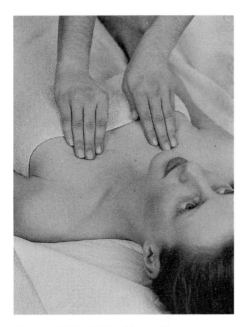

Figure 8.15 Digital kneading to pectoralis major

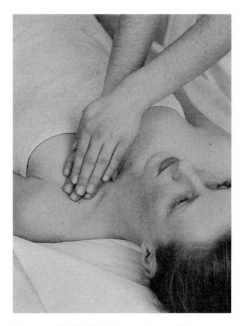

Figure 8.16 Reinforced stroking to the decollete area

DÉCOLLETÉ AREA

- ◆ stroking over area (right hand first, then left hand)
- ◆ effleurage around shoulders and back
- ◆ digital kneading to pectoralis major
- ◆ digital kneading to upper fibres of trapezius on back of shoulders
- ◆ reinforced stroking (figure of eight)
- ◆ effleurage

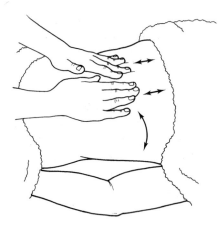

Figure 8.17 Effleurage to abdomen

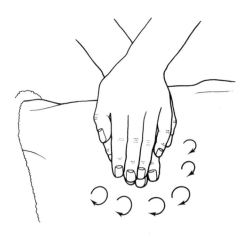

Figure 8.18 Digital kneading to colon

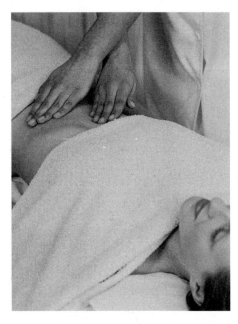

Figure 8.19 Circular kneading to abdomen

ABDOMEN

◆ effleurage

◆ reinforced kneading to the waist

◆ wringing to the waist if suitable

◆ stroking over abdomen

◆ circular kneading around abdomen

◆ digital kneading around colon

◆ ulnar border kneading around colon

◆ stroking to colon

◆ effleurage

Back

BONES

The back contains the following bones:

◆ **vertebral column**: made up of 26 separate bones in five regions – cervical (7), thoracic (12), lumbar (5), sacral (5 fused), coccyx (4 fused)

- ◆ **ribs**: 12 pairs of ribs form the thorax and articulate with the spine behind and the sternum in front

- ◆ **scapulae**: these lie on the upper back, one on each side of the vertebral column

- ◆ **innominate** or **pelvic**: these articulate with the sacrum behind, forming a ring of bone known as the pelvis. They join to form a cartilaginous joint called the symphysis pubis in front.

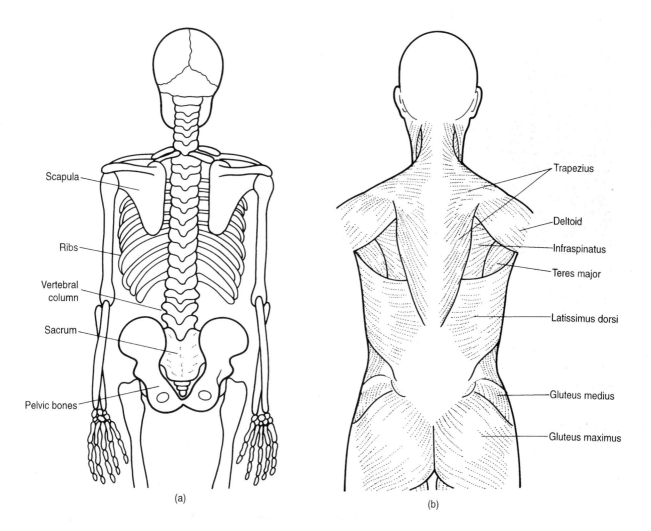

Scapula

Ribs

Vertebral
column

Sacrum

Pelvic bones

(a)

Trapezius

Deltoid

Infraspinatus

Teres major

Latissimus dorsi

Gluteus medius

Gluteus maximus

(b)

Figure 8.20 Anatomy of the back (a) bones (b) muscles

JOINTS

Table 8.7 Classification of back joints

Name	Type	Movement
Intervertebral	Cartilaginous, between the vertebrae	Very little movement between each pair, but considerable movement when spine moves as a whole. Flexion, extension, side flexion and rotation
Sacroiliac	Gliding (synovial) between the sacrum and right and left innominate bones	Hardly any movement; slightly increases during pregnancy

MUSCLES

Table 8.8 Classification of back muscles

Name	Position	Action
Trapezius	Covers the upper back	Extends the head and elevates the shoulders. When one side is working it flexes the head to the same side and elevates one shoulder
Rhomboid major and minor	Lie deep to trapezius between the scapulae	Retract the shoulder girdle
Latissimus dorsi	Covers the lower back. From the lumbar region it passes upwards and outwards and inserts on the front of the humerus	Extends the shoulder joint and medially rotates it. Raises the trunk towards the arms as in climbing
Erector spinae	Lies deep to other muscles. Forms three columns from lumbar spine up along ribs to transverse and spinous processes to the cervical spine	Extends the trunk; one side working, side flexes the trunk to the same side
Quadratus lumborum	Deepest muscle lying on either side of the lumbar spine	Extends the trunk; one side working, side flexes the trunk to the same side

LYMPHATIC DRAINAGE

- ◆ The upper back drains into the axillary nodes.

- ◆ The lower back drains into the inguinal nodes.

POINTS TO CONSIDER

Before commencing massage it is important to examine the client's back carefully as many variations are found.

Observe the spine

- ◆ Is it straight or does it curve to the left or right indicating scoliosis?

- ◆ Is there a humped look in the thoracic region indicating kyphosis? An extra pillow may be required below the bust to improve contour and comfort.

- ◆ Is there a deep hollowing in the lumbar region indicating lordosis? An extra pillow may be required under the abdomen to level out the lumbar spine and improve comfort.

Observe the scapulae

- ◆ Do they lie flat on the thoracic wall or does the medial border and inferior angle protrude backward, indicating winged scapulae?

- ◆ Are the scapulae level or is one higher than the other? This may indicate muscle tension in the upper fibres of the trapezius or it may simply be the way the client is lying – adjust the client's position.

Observe the skin and underlying tissue

- ◆ Are there any skin conditions which would make massage unsuitable (contra-indicated), e.g. extensive or pustular acne, large raised freckling, etc?

Observe and feel the underlying tissues

- ◆ Does one area look raised? Is it hard and tense rather than soft and relaxed to touch? Are there painful, tender areas or nodules?

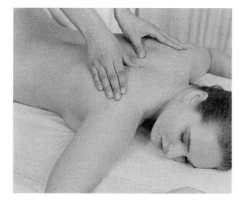

Figure 8.21 Thumb kneading between scapulae

By observation, palpation and sensing through the hands in this way, you will build up a mental picture

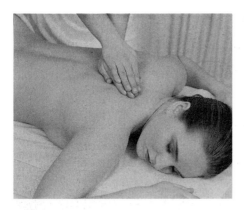

Figure 8.22 Reinforced stroking around scapulae

which will enable you to adapt your massage as necessary, e.g. avoid all bony prominences by working around them away from curve. Tense areas will require a slow, rhythmical, relaxing massage and tension nodules may require frictions. Extra work may be required over the upper and middle fibres of the trapezius. If there is pain in the lumbar region, the massage should be very light and gentle in that area.

MASSAGE ROUTINE

The suggested massage routine for the back is as follows:

◆ stroking over back for palpating and sensing the tissues

◆ effleurage over back

◆ effleurage over trapezius (neck and shoulders)

◆ digital or thumb kneading to upper fibres of trapezius

◆ digital or thumb kneading from neck down between scapulae

◆ circular kneading around scapulae

◆ reinforced stroking around scapulae (figure of eight)

◆ alternate palmar kneading all over back

◆ reinforced kneading to waist

◆ wringing along hip, waist and side of ribs (if suitable)

◆ double-handed kneading over back (one side to other and back in four strips)

◆ transverse stroking over back

◆ thumb kneading to sacrum

◆ digital kneading down right and left erector spinae

◆ stroking down right and left erector spinae

◆ effleurage over back.

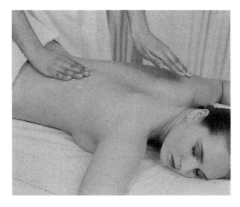

Figure 8.23 Stroking down erector spinae

Light hacking and cupping over the back may be included for an invigorating massage.

?

1 Explain the sequence of a body massage routine.

2 State how effleurage is incorporated into a body massage.

3 Explain how you would adapt depth, speed and rhythm for the following types of massage:

   (a) a relaxing massage

   (b) a general massage

   (c) an invigorating massage.

4 Give the two standing positions used in massage.

5 Name the large group of muscles on:

   (a) the front of the thigh

   (b) the back of the thigh.

6 Explain why it is difficult to perform wringing or picking up on the lateral aspect of the thigh.

7 Name the bony prominences on the leg which must be avoided.

8 Explain why the heavier massage manipulations should *not* be performed over the abdomen.

9 Name two groups of lymph nodes in the leg and two groups in the arm.

10 Explain briefly how you would massage tight, tense muscles across the upper back.

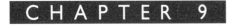

CHAPTER 9

Adapting massage for specific conditions

OBJECTIVES

After you have studied this chapter you will be able to:

1 list the problems and conditions which may benefit from massage
2 explain the importance of psychological preparation prior to a relaxing massage
3 perform a relaxing massage for reduction of stress and tension
4 explain how visual and verbal feedback are obtained from the client
5 perform a massage to combat mental and physical fatigue
6 explain what is meant by the term 'oedema'
7 relate oedema to the function of the lymphatic system
8 select appropriate manipulations for the treatment of oedema
9 perform a massage to relieve oedema
10 describe the nature of cellulite and explain how it differs from soft fat
11 select appropriate manipulations for the treatment of cellulite
12 perform a suitable massage for the treatment of cellulite
13 discuss other treatments which may be used to treat cellulite
14 explain the advice you would give a client to combat cellulite.

Conditions which benefit from massage

During the initial detailed client consultation you will have established why massage is a suitable treatment for the client. The type of massage will vary depending on the desired outcomes of the treatment and on the age, physical and mental condition of the client. It is important to be flexible and adaptable, and to avoid keeping rigidly to set routines. Manipulations and routines must be adapted to suit each client – some manipulations may be omitted while others will be used more extensively. Massage is beneficial for a variety of conditions and problems:

◆ to relieve stress and tension and promote relaxation

◆ to stimulate a lethargic client suffering mental and physical fatigue (to promote alertness)

◆ to relieve muscle fatigue, pain and soreness (post-performance or event)

◆ to relax very painful, stiff muscles

◆ to prepare and warm muscles prior to specific activities (pre-performance or event)

◆ to relieve or reduce areas of oedema (swelling)

◆ to stimulate and soften areas of cellulite

◆ to promote figure awareness during weight loss when used in conjunction with other treatments and diet

◆ to improve digestion and relieve constipation

◆ to improve the condition and tone of the skin

◆ to relieve stress for clients with certain heart and blood pressure conditions

◆ to relieve pain and stiffness in specific areas, particularly in the upper and lower back or to treat fibrositis.

Reducing stress and tension

Before commencing a relaxing massage it is important to prepare the mind as well as the body. The atmosphere created in the working environment must be quiet and calming. The area must be private, warm, well ventilated and free from distracting noises. The client must be positioned in a comfortable, well-supported position. S/he must feel safe and secure.

The therapist should adopt a relaxed, unhurried manner, speaking positively, calmly and quietly. Her/his movements should be smooth and gliding rather than sudden or jerky.

The client must be greeted pleasantly and made to feel cared for and cosseted. The procedure should be clearly explained and the client should be encouraged to ask questions which must be answered immediately. S/he must be encouraged to discuss any problems or worries which may contribute to stress. A sympathetic but not patronising approach will reduce anxiety and help the client to relax. This is particularly important with new or nervous clients. Relaxation can be further encouraged by suggesting that the client empties the mind or concentrates on some pleasant visual imagery. Keep conversation to a minimum once the massage has started. Although most of these factors apply to most massage treatments, they are particularly important for relaxation and will greatly influence the effectiveness of the treatment.

List all the methods you would use to create a suitable atmosphere for promoting mental and physical relaxation.

TREATMENT TECHNIQUE

The massage must be smooth, slow, deep and rhythmical. The transition between strokes should be continuous and barely perceptible. The tempo must be constant and unhurried. All the effleurage and petrissage movements in the suggested routines may be included, but percussion must never be included in a relaxing massage as the movements are too invigorating and stimulating.

You may wish to use more effleurage and kneading manipulations, repeating the movements until you feel the muscles softening and relaxing under your hands. You may need to concentrate and perform more manipulations on specific, identified areas of tension such as around the shoulder region, the upper or lower back or over the large muscle groups of the legs. Slow down each effleurage stroke at the end of the treatment.

Remember that it is very important to work calmly and unhurriedly, with constant, slow rhythm and medium depth. You must maintain your concentration throughout – you should relax mentally and physically as the massage progresses, but keep concentrating.

FEEDBACK AND ADVICE

At the end of the massage you should obtain visual and verbal feedback.

Visual feedback is obtained by looking at the area:

◆ Is there an erythema?

◆ Is it even or patchy?

◆ Do the muscles look and feel softer and more relaxed?

◆ Are there still some tight hard areas?

Verbal feedback is obtained by asking the client some questions:

◆ How did that feel?

◆ Did you go to sleep?

◆ Was any part of the massage uncomfortable?

◆ Did any manipulation irritate or tickle?

◆ Did you want me to spend longer on any area?

◆ Were you able to relax mentally?

From this feedback you will formulate a strategy for the next treatment. Discuss with the client any changes you intend making, giving the reasons why they are needed. Record these on the record card and refer to them next time.

Give the client home advice on reducing stress and practising relaxation techniques. (These techniques can be found in *Body Fitness and Exercise* by Mo Rosser.)

Combating mental and physical fatigue

For this type of client it is very important to create a stimulating atmosphere. Although the therapist must be caring and sympathetic, a positive, cheerful attitude is also required.

During consultation the client should be encouraged to discuss any problems and to establish reasons for the lethargy or tiredness. There are many factors which may cause the condition: stress at work or in the home; feeling overburdened or overworked; insufficient time for rest, relaxation or enjoyment; feeling unwell, suffering with headaches, migraine, insomnia or heavy and prolonged periods. There may also be psychological problems such as unhappiness, depression, feelings of low esteem or lack of achievement, etc.

Encourage the client to seek solutions to the problems through changes in lifestyle, or to see a doctor if ill health is a cause.

> *List other reasons why clients may feel fatigued and lethargic.*

TREATMENT TECHNIQUE

Treatment for this type of client will be similar to that of a general massage. However, certain adaptations should be made. The massage movements will again be smooth, deep and rhythmical, but of moderate to brisk speed. The speed of the effleurage strokes may be increased with each movement. This is particularly important at the end of the treatment as it stimulates alertness. Note the difference from a relaxing or general massage, where the speed slows down towards the last stroke.

Petrissage movements should be deep and brisk. Light tapotement movements should also be included, unless there are contra-indications. These hacking and cupping movements are invigorating and may be performed over the quadriceps muscles, the calf, the hamstrings, the buttocks, and very lightly over the top of the shoulders and along the back. Make sure that the client has a reasonable covering of flesh over the ribs and is not too thin or tapotement will be painful and contra-indicated. Frictions performed along either side of the spinal column are also very effective as they stimulate the spinal nerves. Complete the massage with brisk effleurage.

FEEDBACK AND ADVICE

Obtain visual and verbal feedback.

Visual feedback

◆ Is there a good even erythema?

◆ Are there any very red or sore spots indicating over-treatment?

◆ Does the client seem more alert?

◆ Is the client satisfied with the treatment; is s/he happy and smiling?

Verbal feedback

◆ How did that feel?

◆ Was there any discomfort; did it hurt anywhere?

◆ Did you enjoy it?

◆ Did you want more treatment on any particular area?

Discuss and plan the strategy for next time. Give home advice as appropriate. For example, you might suggest that the client should try to reduce her/his workload, allow time for rest, practise relaxation techniques, go to bed early some nights of the week, relax with a bath, and make time for enjoyment.

Relieving oedema

It is important to understand the structure and function of the lymphatic system before practising this massage (see Chapter 2).

Oedema is swelling of the tissues due to an accumulation and stagnation of tissue fluid in tissue spaces. Normally this tissue fluid is drained away through the blood vessels or lymphatic vessels. If these systems fail to drain the fluid away, it will remain in the tissue spaces. The amount of swelling can vary from slight puffiness, to soft, mobile swelling which yields easily to pressure, or hard, consolidated, unyielding swelling of long standing. There are many possible causes of oedema:

◆ obstruction or blockage of the lymphatic system, such as an infected node

◆ interference in part of the system following surgery where glands may have been removed

◆ increase in the permeability of blood vessel walls or pressure within the vessels forcing fluid out. If this excess fluid cannot be removed quickly enough by the lymphatic system it remains in the tissue spaces

◆ lack of muscle contraction which acts as a pump and assists blood and lymphatic flow

◆ standing for long periods so that gravitational pull and lack of muscle contraction slow lymphatic drainage of the leg. Fluid collects around the ankle which becomes puffy and swollen. The legs will feel tired and heavy.

Because massage speeds up the flow of blood in the veins and the flow of lymph in the lymph vessels, it is a useful treatment in the prevention and reduction of oedema. A brisk general or leg massage will be effective if oedema is recent, soft and due to gravitational effects. However, special techniques must be used if the oedema is of long standing, hard and consolidated, and the covering skin is shiny, thin and stretched. Great care must be taken not to break or damage the skin.

A squeezing movement is used to apply and then release pressure along the path of lymphatic flow. This alternating pressure technique forces the fluid out of the tissue spaces and speeds flow through the lymphatic vessels. It is important to drain and clear the proximal end first (i.e. the part nearest the lymph nodes). This ensures that fluid is not pushed into an already engorged area. The part must be elevated so that gravity assists the flow. Squeezing, kneading, effleurage and vibrations are the manipulations used.

TREATMENT TECHNIQUE

OEDEMATOUS LEG

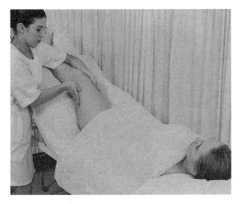

Figure 9.1 Position of client with leg in elevation

1 Prepare the client as for a general massage. Make sure that all restrictive clothing is removed and that there is no tight elastic if underwear is not removed.

2 Place the client in the supine position (face up). Make sure that the legs lie on the elevating end of the couch.

3 Elevate the leg to 45° from the horizontal by raising the end of the bed if possible, or by using an arrangement of firm pillows.

4 The legs must be allowed to drain in this position for half to one hour (you may massage other areas during this time). Massaging the abdomen can increase the effectiveness of the following leg massage. This is because lymph flow through the abdominal vessels, iliac nodes and lymph ducts is stimulated and drained away, reducing backward pressure. Deep breathing is also beneficial because as the client breathes in and out the pressure within the thoracic and abdominal cavities increases and decreases. The alternating high to low pressure acts as a pump, moving fluid along; this also reduces backward pressure.

5 Examine the leg carefully before starting the massage. Check the skin and the degree of hardness of the oedema (does it 'pit' easily under pressure and refill quickly or slowly). This will give some indication of how much pressure can be applied. If it is hard and unyielding, start with lighter pressure.

6 Take up a walk standing stance, level with the knee.

7 Imagine that you are pushing fluid through a tube or many tubes. To be effective, pressure must be applied to all the surfaces of the tube.

8 Begin just below the inguinal nodes in the groin. With one hand on the inner leg and the other on the outer side, cover as much of the circumference as possible; now squeeze inward and upward, four to six times.

9 Now place one hand on the front and one on the back and squeeze in an upward direction, four to six times.

10 Repeat this squeezing until the area softens.

11 As you feel the area softening slightly, perform small circular palmar kneading movements over the area (both palms pressing together). Cover the sides, front and back thoroughly.

12 Next, effleurage slowly towards the groin.

13 Move the hands down the leg, one hand width only at a time, overlapping the previous area. Repeat the above manipulations. Work gently and slowly in this way until you reach the knee.

14 Now perform palmar kneading then effleurage over the entire thigh. As the tissues soften, deeper pressure may be applied and larger movements performed.

15 Move below the knee to drain the lower leg into the popliteal nodes. Begin just below the knee.

16 Avoid the anterior border of the tibia (shin bone). Cup the hands around the calf with the heels of the hands on either side of the shin bone. Squeeze in and upwards until the oedema softens. Vibrate the hands in and out. Knead the calf then effleurage.

17 Work gradually down the leg, one hand width at a time.

18 Work thoroughly around the ankles as fluid frequently stagnates around the medial and lateral malleoli.

19 Cup one hand behind the ankle joint – the thumb and thenar eminence on one side and the fingers on the other side of the Achilles' tendon. Place the other hand across the front of the joint.

20 Squeeze all the areas together in a pumping and

upward push manner until the tissues soften. Work around the malleoli with the pads of the index, middle and ring fingers. Make small pressure circles around the bones. Then, with the fingers on either side of the Achilles' tendon, push in and up.

21 Press and knead the sole and dorsum of the foot with single-handed kneading.

22 Effleurage the lower leg again.

23 Effleurage the entire leg to complete the massage.

After the massage, active muscle contractions should be performed to exert a pumping action:

◆ pull foot up and down very slowly

◆ turn foot in and out

◆ circle foot around slowly

◆ tighten the quadriceps by pressing the back of the knee into the pillow and pulling the knee cap towards the groin

◆ repeat these movements 10–15 times.

OEDEMATOUS ARM

The following routine is used to promote drainage of the upper arm into the axillary nodes.

1 Elevate the arm to 45° or over – this is usually done with the client sitting on a chair, with the arm supported on a pillow on the elevated end of a plinth. Allow half to one hour for drainage.

2 Begin just below the axilla. Circle the arm with the hand – left hand underneath with fingers pointing medially, right hand over the top with fingers pointing laterally. Squeeze the tissues with inward and upward pressure. As the tissues soften, move the hands distally and overlap slightly. Repeat the squeezing down to the elbow.

3 Follow this with circular kneading over triceps and biceps. Place one hand on the triceps and the other on the biceps, then knead using small circles from the proximal to the distal end.

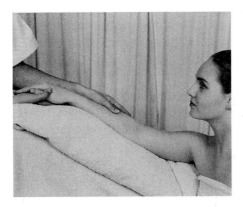

Figure 9.2 Position of client with arm in elevation

4 Effleurage the upper arm: begin proximally, push to axilla, return a hand width further down and push up again to axilla. Continue in this way until the hands reach the elbow.

For drainage of the forearm, repeat the above procedure covering the area from the elbow to the wrist.

OEDEMATOUS HAND

1 Place your left hand vertically behind the client's hand, and your right hand across the palm. Make small circular kneading movements with the palm into the client's palm.

2 Squeeze each finger and thumb gently.

3 Teach active movements of all joints of wrist, hand and elbow.

Reducing cellulite

Cellulite is a condition, found predominantly in women, where areas of adipose tissue (fat) become hard and lumpy and very difficult to remove.

In women cellulite is found mainly on the outer thighs, hips and buttocks, abdomen, midriff and back of the arms. In men it is usually distributed around the waist. It is more common and more widely distributed in the female because of the greater amount of oestrogen produced. This hormone encourages the laying down of fat.

The areas of cellulite look dimpled or lumpy, and feel hard and cold to touch. Pushing the flesh between the hands makes the skin very uneven and puckered, similar to the surface of orange peel.

Cellulite is more commonly found in overweight individuals, but is also found in slim people and those of ideal weight. In the slim it is present in specific areas, usually the outer thighs, giving the characteristic 'jodhpur' shape. Cellulite is difficult to reduce and remove, even when the individual is on a reducing diet and exercising regularly. Research indicates that there is no physiological difference between cellulite and the more easily removed fat, but there are differences in the supporting connective tissue and in the organisation and circulation of the subcutaneous tissues in cellulitic areas.

The body stores fat for use as fuel when required. The digestive system breaks down the food we eat to provide energy for bodily functions. If the energy input is greater than the energy output (i.e. if we eat more food than is required for energy), then the excess fuel is stored in the body as fat.

Fat is stored in specialised cells called **adipocytes**. These form clusters supported by connective tissue, which group together to form adipose tissue. This is found under the skin in the subcutaneous layer, and among muscle fibres around organs such as the kidneys and heart. Complex chemical reactions convert the food eaten into fat for storage, and again from storage to use as fuel for energy. Although fat will be used from areas all over the body when required, it appears to be more difficult to remove from certain areas. These areas of hard, difficult-to-remove fat are called cellulite.

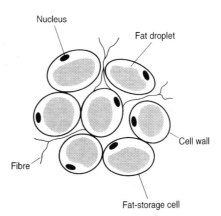

Figure 9.3 Storage of fat in adipocytes

In cellulitic areas there is some alteration of the subcutaneous tissue. The adipocytes become overloaded and develop a tough outer membrane. The supporting connective tissue increases, enmeshing groups of adipocytes together in a lobular structure. This gives the dimpled, uneven appearance of the area.

The overloaded cells and lobules compress the capillary networks and lymphatics. This interferes with the circulation to the area. Stagnation and deficient circulation adversely affect the area: the tissues do not receive the required nutrients and oxygen; waste products (toxins) accumulate in the area as they are not quickly removed; and the temperature of the area will be lowered as warm blood is not circulating normally (hence it feels cold to touch). Fat remains in the overloaded adipocytes as it is not easily removed by the poorly circulating blood for conversion to energy, and the area becomes hard and stagnated. If action is not taken, the condition will become progressively worse, with greater engorgement of the area, degeneration of connective tissue and hardening of the fatty tissue.

TREATMENT TECHNIQUES

The aims of the treatment are:

1 to soften and reduce the fatty adipose layer

2 to increase the circulation to the area, thus improving nutrition

3 to speed up blood and lymphatic drainage from the area, thus removing toxins more quickly

4 to improve the condition of the skin.

Successful treatment will involve combining a variety of treatments into an effective routine, which will include both manual and mechanical massage.

It is important to remember that spot reduction of fat from a specific area is not possible. To reduce body fat, calorie intake must be less than calorie output. Only then is fat removed from body stores and broken down for energy. The clients must therefore be given advice on sensible eating and made aware of the factors which are thought to contribute to cellulite (see 'advice to clients', on page 149).

A variety of treatments may be used to combat cellulite, but massage should always complete the treatment to improve drainage.

ELECTRICAL TREATMENTS

◆ **Electrical muscle stimulation** (EMS) to underlying muscles is effective because as the muscles contract and relax they exert a pumping action on the blood and lymphatic vessels. This stimulates the circulation in the deeper tissues and the metabolic rate of the area is improved. The sensory nerve endings in the skin will be stimulated and this will produce reflex dilation of the capillaries in the dermis, increasing blood flow to and from the area.

◆ **Galvanic treatment**, using the cathode over the area of cellulite, produces the alkali sodium hydroxide which will soften the skin and tissues. It results in vasodilatation with hyperaemia and erythema, so more blood flows to and from the area. Water molecules are drawn towards the cathode which will soften the area. Various anti-cellulite products containing negatively charged ions will be repelled by the cathode into the skin. These are designed to break down and aid the dispersal of cellulite.

◆ **Specialised body systems** using body wraps, clays, serums, creams and low-intensity currents are effective in stimulating the circulation.

◆ **Vacuum suction** is effective as it speeds up lymphatic and venous drainage of the area, removing fluid and toxins. Cups with reduced pressure are moved over the area in the direction of lymphatic drainage towards the nearest set of lymph nodes. The suction dilates the vessels as the cup moves along, increasing flow. Vacuum suction is effective after EMS and mechanical massage (G5). If combined with galvanic treatment it should be given first to decongest the area. Do not use massage or vacuum suction after galvanic treatment as the areas under the pads are too sensitive.

◆ **Mechanical massage** (G5) produces a deeper effect and more stimulation of the body tissues than manual massage. The spiky head will stimulate and increase the circulation to the skin, producing an erythema. The increase in the delivery of nutrients and oxygen, the removal of waste products (metabolites), the increase in metabolic rate and the desquamating effect will all improve the condition of the skin. The deep kneading movements, using the 'eggbox' or hard spiked rubber heads, will affect the deeper tissues. The pressure of the strokes must be directed upwards to aid venous and lymphatic drainage. This massage warms and softens the area and speeds up the removal of metabolites. Heavy kneading movements should be brisk but not too prolonged, as resulting dilation of capillaries and blood vessels may increase the fluid in the area further, engorging it and increasing compression.

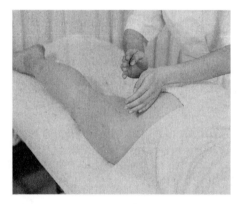

Figure 9.4 Hacking over the buttocks

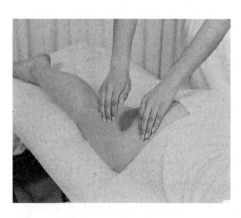

Figure 9.5 Cupping over the buttocks

MANUAL MASSAGE

This forms an important part of the treatment and should conclude the treatment plan. As with mechanical massage, all manipulations must follow the direction of venous return and lymphatic drainage. As the flow in these vessels is speeded up, fluid and metabolites from tissue cells and spaces are removed more efficiently, reducing stagnation (stasis). The arterial circulation will in turn increase, bringing nutrients and oxygen to nourish the tissues, and the metabolic rate will increase. This improves the stagnant area. It may be that fat needed for fuel will be mobilised from this stimulated area, but there is no scientific research evidence to prove this.

The heavier manipulations of kneading, picking up, wringing, hacking, cupping, beating and pounding may be used over the areas of cellulite, according to client needs. The greater the depth and the more consolidated and harder the cellulite, the deeper the manipulations should be. Deep, brisk effleurage along the length of the area should conclude the massage.

If galvanic treatment has been used, remember that the area under the pads will be very sensitive. Therefore massage may be given proximal to (above) the area and around the padded areas to conclude the treatment.

ADVICE TO CLIENTS

It is important that clients are made aware of the factors which are thought to contribute to the build up of cellulite. They should be encouraged to follow a self-help, daily regime which will increase the efficiency of the treatment. The following home advice should be given.

1 Eat a well-balanced diet:

- ◆ include all the nutrients necessary for health, i.e. a little fat, proteins, carbohydrates, vitamins, minerals, water and fibre

- ◆ eat plenty of fresh fruit and vegetables (five portions a day are recommended); do not overcook vegetables

- ◆ eat oily fish such as herring, trout, mackerel, and salmon

- ◆ eat wholemeal foods such as wholemeal bread, pasta, rice, cereals, pulses and beans

- ◆ reduce intake of saturated fat found in butter, dairy products and red meat

- ◆ reduce intake of sugar and salt

- ◆ reduce intake of alcohol – 7 to 14 units per week only

- ◆ drink around 3 litres of water per day.

2 Balance energy intake with energy output:

- ◆ if the diet provides just enough energy to meet body requirements, there is no surplus to be stored, therefore no fat to be deposited. To reduce fatty tissue, energy input must be less than energy output. Only then will fat be utilised from body stores to provide required fuel

- ◆ reducing the diet and increasing aerobic activity is the best regime for reducing fat (e.g. walking, jogging, swimming or cycling for 20–30 minutes, twice to three times per week, is excellent).

3 Avoid wearing tight clothes that apply pressure and restrict the circulation, such as tight jeans or trousers, tight belts, underwear and corsets.

4 Take plenty of exercise and keep mobile during the day. If in a sedentary occupation, it is advisable to walk around, swing the legs and stretch at regular intervals.

5 Breath correctly and deeply:

♦ practise deep breathing, thus using all areas of the lungs. Breath in deeply and feel the sternum move forwards, the ribs move outwards and the diaphragm move downwards, pushing the abdomen out. Breath out and feel the sternum move back, the ribs move in and down and the abdomen pull in

♦ when sitting or lying, breathing is shallow and uses mainly the upper chest. Deep breathing uses the chest capacity to the full and increases the intake of oxygen. The alternating pressure in the thoracic and abdominal cavities also stimulates the circulation around the body.

6 Eat plenty of roughage and drink 2–3 litres of water per day. This will aid digestion, prevent constipation and facilitate the elimination of waste products from the body.

Male clients

The male client must be received with the same polite, caring manner as the female. As always, the highest standards of professionalism apply. Avoid bantering and ignore any suggestive comments or innuendo.

TREATMENT TECHNIQUE

PREPARATION

1 Before the client undresses give clear instructions on use of the shower and covering towels, the return to the massage area and the positioning on the bed. Brief pants can be worn throughout the massage.

2 Position the towel widthways across the chest. Place a folded towel (double layer) across the lower abdomen. Place another towel lengthways over the previous towel and over the legs.

3 Men are frequently hairy and massage may be uncomfortable if insufficient oil or talcum powder is used. Talcum powder is often a better medium over hairy areas – apply liberally. If oil is used, ensure that it is not too viscous and again apply liberally.

ADAPTATION OF STROKES

1 Men generally have denser, firmer and larger muscles than women, depending on their degree of fitness. Massage manipulations may therefore be deeper and heavier, but this must be adapted to suit each client.

2 Stroking manipulations may be performed in the direction of hair growth, usually downwards. These movements should be light.

3 Effleurage should be performed in the direction of venous return, using plenty of oil or talcum powder. (If this pulls against the direction of hair growth or is uncomfortable, omit the movement.)

4 Petrissage manipulations also require care and a liberal amount of the massage medium.

5 More percussion manipulations may be included unless the client requires a relaxing massage.

6 Cover the body parts in the following order, omitting the abdomen:

◆ front of legs (avoiding the femoral triangle)

◆ arms – work over side of chest can be included with each arm

◆ back of legs

◆ back.

Where a male therapist is required to give massage to a female client, the chest and abdomen areas are omitted from the routine.

?

1 List six conditions or problems which will benefit from massage.

2 Explain why it is important for the treatment room to be warm, well ventilated and quiet.

3 Give three important considerations of technique when giving massage for relaxation.

4 Explain what is meant by the following:

   (a) visual feedback

   (b) verbal feedback.

5 List six reasons why clients may feel tired and lethargic.

6 Give two manipulations that may be used for invigorating a tired client that would not be used in a relaxing massage.

7 Explain why the part should be elevated when giving massage to relieve oedema.

8 Explain why movements for relieving oedema should begin proximally and not distally as in a general massage.

9 Give the three main movements used when treating oedema.

10 Describe the appearance of cellulite.

11 Give two areas of the body where cellulite is found in women.

12 Give four aims of treatment when dealing with cellulite.

13 List two other treatments which may be used in conjunction with massage for the treatment of cellulite.

14 Explain why care must be taken when using massage following galvanic treatments.

15 Explain briefly the home advice you would give a client who wished to reduce areas of cellulite.

16 Explain how you would adapt the massage for a male client.

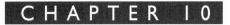

Mechanical massage

· ·

OBJECTIVES

After you have studied this chapter you will be able to:

1 distinguish between the different types of mechanical massage equipment
2 distinguish between the effects produced by the different types of equipment and the various 'heads'
3 select the appropriate massage equipment to suit the needs of the client
4 identify any contra-indications to the treatment
5 treat the client, paying due consideration to maximum efficiency, comfort, safety and hygiene.

Mechanical massage is the manipulation of body tissues using machines. Generally, mechanical massage is used in conjunction with other treatments to relieve muscle tension and muscle pain, to improve the circulation and to improve certain skin conditions. Provided the client is on a reducing diet, the heavier vibrations may help to disperse fatty deposits from specific areas of the body.

Many different types of appliance are manufactured to produce effects similar to those of a manual massage. They vary from the small hand-held percussion and audio-sonic equipment designed to treat small, localised areas, to the large heavy gyratory vibrators used for deeper effects on large areas of the body. Although the effects are similar to those of manual massage, the sensation felt by the client is very different. The treatment is rather impersonal and the use of a machine rather than the touch of hands is not as pleasing to the client.

In practice, most mechanical vibratory treatments should be combined with some manual massage, thus gaining the more personal aspects of manual massage combined with the depth and power of vibratory equipment. Using mechanical massage equipment is certainly less tiring for the therapist than performing a long, vigorous manual massage. The effects produced are similar for all types of massage equipment, but are deeper and greater with the heavier machines. The treatment is very popular with clients as they feel invigorated and consider that the desired results will be achieved.

Gyratory vibrator

Massage with this type of appliance is much heavier than with percussion and audio-sonic vibrators. It is therefore more suitable for heavier work on large and bulky areas of the body. There are two main types of appliance.

1 **The hand-held vibrator**: this is heavy to use as all the electrical component parts are held in the hand. It is useful for domiciliary work.

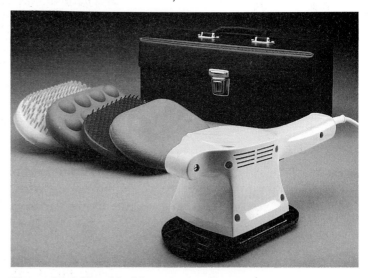

Figure 10.1 Hand-held gyratory vibrator

2 **The floor-standing vibrator**, commonly called G5: this is a very popular treatment in the salon. Here all the electrical components are housed in a box which is supported by a stand, and only the moving

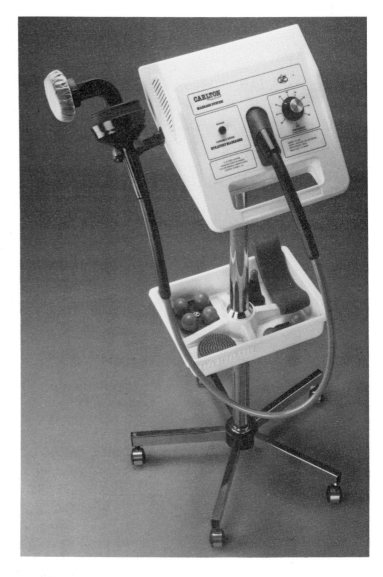

Figure 10.2 Floor-standing gyratory vibrator

head is held in the hand. This machine uses a rotary electric motor to turn a crank, which is attached to the head. The head is driven to turn in gyratory motion, moving round and round, up and down and side to side with pressure, providing a deep massage. A variety of attachments is available, which screw onto the head; they are designed to stimulate the movements of manual massage:

(a) effleurage: sponge heads, curved and disc

(b) petrissage: hard rubber heads, single and

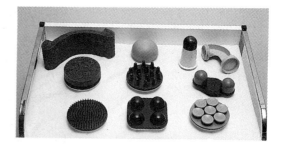

Figure 10.3 Examples of different heads for the gyratory vibrator

double ball, flat disc, four half-ball (eggbox), multi-hard spike

(c) tapotement: fine spiky and brush heads.

TREATMENT TECHNIQUE

PREPARATION OF THE CLIENT

1 Place the client in a well-supported comfortable position.

2 Check that all jewellery has been removed.

3 Check for contra-indications.

4 Clean the skin with cologne.

5 Explain the treatment to the client.

6 Select the appropriate pre-heating treatment.

7 Apply talcum powder to the area using effleurage strokes (do not use oil as it may cause deterioration of the sponge heads).

PROCEDURE

1 Select the appropriate heads to suit the needs of the client. Do not change the heads too often as this breaks the continuity of the treatment.

(a) **Effleurage:** use curved sponge on limbs or round sponge elsewhere.

(b) **Kneading:** use the flat disc head for lighter petrissage; the four-ball head for deeper petrissage; the multi, large spike for very deep petrissage on very heavy areas of adipose tissue;

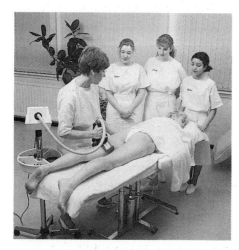

Figure 10.4 Demonstration of treatment using gyratory vibrator

and the single and double ball heads on specific, localised areas.

(c) **Desquamation:** use fine spiky and brush heads.

To maintain high standards of hygiene, the heads can be placed in a plastic bag, which should be changed for each client.

2 Switch the machine on, holding the head below the level of the couch. (This is a safety precaution in case the head is insecure – if it flies off it will not hit the client.)

3 With the sponge applicator, apply in long sweeping strokes following the direction of venous return and natural contours of the body. The stroke should be light and smooth rather than abrupt and jerky. The pressure should be heavier on muscle bulk. Cover the area well.

4 Change the head for kneading. Use a circular kneading motion, using the other hand to support the tissues and lift them towards the head. Again apply upward pressure and work with venous return. Cover the area well.

5 Keep the surface of the attachment parallel to the surface of the body at all times. (If one side lifts off the body, there is a danger of damaging the tissues with the hard edge of the head.)

6 Change to the effleurage head to complete the treatment.

7 The degree of erythema and client tolerance dictates the length of the treatment.

8 Wash the heads in hot water and detergent, and allow them to dry.

Note: particular care should be taken when selecting heads for treating the abdominal wall. Abdominal organs have no bony framework for protection – their only protection is provided by the muscles and tissues of the abdominal wall. Over-stretched muscles with poor tone offer less protection. This must be considered when treating the abdomen. The heavier petrissage heads should only be used on well-toned abdominal muscles with a covering of adipose tissue, e.g. the younger, overweight client.

EFFECTS

1 As with manual massage, the main effect is stimulation of the circulation. The movements speed up the flow of blood in the veins, removing deoxygenated blood and waste products more rapidly. This affects the arterial circulation, bringing oxygenated blood and nutrients to the area. Lymph drainage via the lymphatic vessels is also increased.

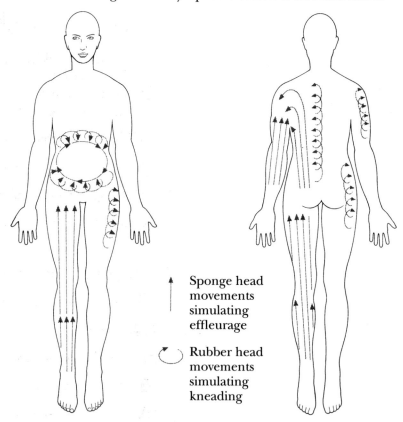

Sponge head movements simulating effleurage

Rubber head movements simulating kneading

Figure 10.5 Direction of strokes for gyratory vibrator

2 Increased blood supply will increase the metabolic rate in the tissues. This will improve the condition of the tissues.

3 Increased blood supply and friction of the heads will raise the temperature of the area and therefore aid muscle relaxation and relieve pain.

4 Pain in muscles may also be relieved due to rapid removal of waste products, such as lactic acid.

5 Surface capillaries dilate giving an erythema. This improves skin tone.

6 The desquamating effect of the heads may improve the texture of the skin.

7 The continuous heavy pressure on adipose tissue and increased circulation to the area may aid the dispersion of fatty deposits if the client is on a reducing diet.

USES

The gyratory vibrator is used:

1 for spot reduction of fatty deposits in conjunction with other treatments and reduced food intake

2 to relieve muscular tension

3 to reduce muscular aches and pains

4 to improve poor circulation

5 to improve the texture of dry, flaky, rough skin.

CONTRA-INDICATIONS

1 skin diseases and disorders

2 bruises

3 dilated capillaries

4 varicose veins

5 thrombosis or phlebitis

6 skin tags, warts or pigmented moles

7 recent operations and scar tissue

8 treatment of the abdomen during pregnancy and menstruation

9 extremely hairy areas

10 thin, bony clients

elderly clients with thin, crêpey skin and lack of subcutaneous fat

12 acute back and spinal problems, e.g. disc trouble

DANGERS

Heavy and prolonged treatments can cause bruising and dilated capillaries.

PRECAUTIONS

1 Check for contra-indications.
2 Do not use heavy percussion over bony areas or over the abdomen with poor muscle tone.
3 Do not over-treat one area, keep the head moving.
4 Keep the head surface parallel to the surface of the body and adapt to body contours.
5 Hold the head away from the client when switching on in case the head is insecure and becomes detached. Hold the head below the bed for safety.
6 Cover the heads with a plastic bag, which can be changed for each client, for hygienic reasons.

Percussion vibrator

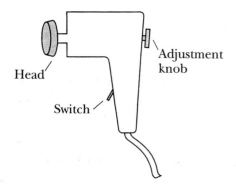

Figure 10.6 Percussion vibrator

This is a hand-held appliance; it is lightweight, easy to use and transport. As its name suggests, it is similar in effect to manual percussion movements. An electric motor is used to make the head move or tap up and down on the skin. The head can be fitted with a variety of attachments, e.g. sponge or spike. Some percussion vibrators have an adjustment knob for increasing and decreasing the intensity of the tap. As the knob is tightened, the tap intensity decreases; as the knob is released, the tap intensity increases. This should be carefully controlled to suit the tissues being treated. The number of movements per second is constant, relating to the frequency of the current. With mains frequency of 50 Hz (cycles per second), each tap occurs every half cycle, therefore the rate of tapping will be 100 per second. The treatment time may vary from 5–15 minutes depending on the desired effects. It is used mainly on the face, neck and across the shoulders.

Audio-sonic vibrator

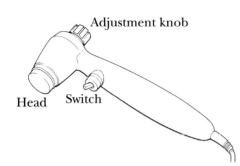

Adjustment knob

Head   Switch

Figure 10.7 Audio-sonic vibrator

This is another type of hand-held appliance. Its name is derived from the fact that the machine produces a humming sound (it should not be confused with ultra-sound therapy, which is quite different). This vibrator uses an electromagnet. When the current is passing one way, the coil moves forward; as the current reverses, the coil moves back. This movement forward and backward is transmitted to the head of the appliance. When the head is placed on the tissues, the forward-backward movement of the coil alternately compresses and decompresses the tissues.

Because the head does not physically move forward and backward, this appliance has a gentler action than the percussion vibrator. It penetrates more deeply into the tissues, but is less stimulating on the surface of the skin. It is, therefore, more suitable for use on sensitive areas of the face and on a mature skin. It is particularly useful for relaxing tension nodules.

TREATMENT TECHNIQUE FOR PERCUSSION AND AUDIO-SONIC VIBRATORS

PREPARATION OF THE CLIENT

1 Place the client in a well-supported and comfortable position.

2 Check that all jewellery has been removed.

3 Check for contra-indications.

4 Explain the treatment to the client.

5 Cleanse the skin.

6 Apply talcum powder for oily/normal skin or cream for dry skin. (Read the manufacturer's instructions.)

PROCEDURE

1 Select the appropriate head and secure it firmly to the vibrator.

2 Switch the machine on away from the client.

3 Commence the treatment using straight lines or a circular motion; ensure coverage of all areas, but avoid delicate areas around the eyes and prominent cheek-bones.

4 The skin reaction indicates the length of the treatment time. When an even erythema is produced, the treatment should stop. This may take from 5 to 15 minutes.

5 The vibrator can be used indirectly over bony or sensitive areas, e.g. cheek-bones and forehead. The therapist places her/his hand between the face and the vibrator head. This reduces the stimulation.

6 Remove the talcum powder or cream and complete the facial routine.

7 Clean the heads, wash with hot water and detergent and disinfect with surgical wipes. Brushes and sponges may be soaked in disinfectant.

EFFECTS

1 It produces an increase in circulation to the treated area, bringing nutrients and oxygen to the area and removing waste products. This improves the condition of the tissues.

2 It produces vasodilation, giving hyperaemia and erythema, improving the colour and tone of the skin.

3 It increases the metabolic rate, thus improving the condition of the tissues.

4 The increase in circulation and the friction of the heads raises the temperature of the area. This promotes relaxation, relieves pain and may stimulate the activity of sebaceous glands.

5 The friction of the heads aids desquamation; this removes the surface layer of cells, improving the condition of the skin.

USES

Percussion and audio-sonic vibrators are used:

1 to stimulate dry, dehydrated or mature skin; the

improved circulation and increase in metabolic rate will improve the condition of the skin

2 to stimulate sebaceous glands; the warmth generated in the tissues will stimulate the production and release of sebum, which will help to lubricate the dry, tired, mature skin

3 to aid desquamation of a sluggish skin; the friction of the heads on the body part will aid the removal of the surface layer, improving texture of the skin

4 to improve and maintain the condition of normal skin

5 to promote relaxation of muscle fibres; the warmth produced in the area will aid relaxation and relieve tension. It is particularly effective over localised tension nodules.

CONTRA-INDICATIONS

1 any skin diseases or inflammatory disorders

2 infected acne

3 highly vascular or telangiectic skin or dilated capillaries

4 sinus problems

5 headaches or migraines

6 lean bony features

7 mature skin with poor elasticity

PRECAUTIONS

1 Check for contra-indications.

2 Do not use over very bony areas.

3 Avoid the eye region.

4 Keep the head surface parallel to the surface of the face.

5 Do not over-treat one area – keep the head moving.

Belt massager

These are usually made of canvas strapping; some have small, ball-like studding in the strapping. The belt is positioned around the area to be treated and the motor moves it back and forth with vibratory motion.

It is generally used to aid the dispersal of fat (provided that the client is on a diet) around the waist, hips and thighs.

?

1 Give three uses for mechanical massage on the body.

2 Name three different types of mechanical massage equipment.

3 List four contra-indications to mechanical massage on the body.

4 List the effects of mechanical massage on the body.

5 Explain briefly why audio-sonic vibrators have an advantage over percussion vibrators on a sensitive area.

6 Give four effects of percussion vibrator treatment to the face.

7 Give two different uses for each of the following:

(a) gyratory vibrator (G5)

(b) percussion vibrator

(c) audio-sonic vibrator.

8 Explain briefly how you would incorporate mechanical massage into a body treatment routine.

9 Give reasons why the heavy gyratory vibrator heads should not be used on the abdominal wall of certain clients.

10 Explain the procedure for maintaining high standards of hygiene when using gyratory vibrators.

CHAPTER 11

Introduction to sports massage

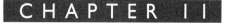

OBJECTIVES

After you have studied this chapter you will be able to:

1 explain the benefits of sports massage
2 list the four categories where massage is used in sport
3 explain the objectives of each category
4 perform the suggested techniques for each category
5 explain the effects of the massage routines in each category.

The field of sport or athletic massage is highly specialised and should not be undertaken by anyone without appropriate training. A qualification in massage is not enough. Additional knowledge and practice under the supervision of an experienced sports massage therapist is required. Further study of anatomy and physiology, with particular emphasis on those systems affected by exercise, is needed. A study of kinesiology (body movement), biomechanics (scientific principles relating to movement) and an understanding of the requirements of the different sports or athletic activities are also necessary.

This in-depth knowledge and understanding will enable the massage therapist to carry out an assessment and provide appropriate treatment for the wide variety of conditions which s/he will encounter. To be effective, the therapist must have empathy and rapport with the performer and the coach or trainer. S/he must be part of the training team, giving advice and explaining the effects and benefits of massage as appropriate. The therapist's knowledge and professionalism must inspire confidence.

Training

Athletes or sportspeople are highly trained, finely tuned individuals who are usually totally focused on achieving success in their particular field. They will train and stress the body to its limit, i.e. to the point of breakdown. They may train too hard and too frequently in an effort to improve performance. Hard training with inadequate rest periods to allow full recovery will result in a decline in performance and leave the body vulnerable to serious injury.

As a result of over-training and incomplete recovery, the athlete may suffer from any of the following symptoms: vague aches and pains; acute pain in muscles, bones or joints; inflammation of tendons, ligaments or bursae resulting in pain and swellings; and symptoms of stress such as headaches, listlessness, tension, insomnia or increased irritability.

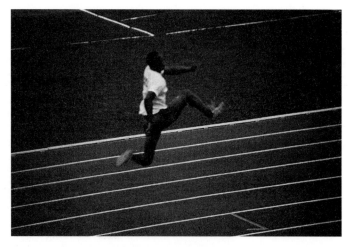

Figure 11.1 A highly-trained athlete

Athletes and their trainers should be made aware that hard training must be balanced with rest periods to allow adequate or full recovery of the tissues and to restore homeostasis (body balance). The harder and longer the training, the longer the rest period should be. If homeostasis is not restored and tissue recovery is incomplete, then the level of performance will eventually decline. Massage following training and performance will greatly hasten the recovery of the tissues. Research indicates that recovery is four to five times faster in tissues receiving massage than in those simply allowed to rest. A shorter recovery time allows for a greater number of training sessions, which will improve performance.

Injuries of the musculo-skeletal system occur as a result of poor technique and over-training. When tired and over-stressed, these structures are more vulnerable to injury. Minor injuries may result in greater injury or serious damage if ignored or neglected. The massage therapist will detect areas of tension and abnormalities within the tissues. Appropriate treatment and rest in these initial stages will prevent further damage.

When injuries occur, they must be referred to a medical practitioner for accurate diagnosis and appropriate treatment. The rate of recovery and return to full function will depend on these factors. Inappropriate treatment or inadequate recovery time may result in further damage and permanently impaired function.

Benefits of sports massage

1. Massage increases the blood flow through the area being massaged, i.e. it produces hyperaemia. The delivery of nutrients and oxygen is therefore increased. These are required for muscle contraction and also to aid recovery of the muscles and maintain them in good condition.

2. Massage generates heat in the tissues through the friction of the hands moving over the surface; through the friction between the tissues as they move over one another; through the dilation of vessels and capillaries which allows more warm blood to flow through the part. Warmth increases the metabolic rate which will improve the condition of the tissues. Warmth also improves flexibility of the tissues, muscle fibres, fascia, tendons and ligaments which are therefore less prone to strains and sprains. Warm muscles contract more efficiently than cold muscles.

3 Deep massage movements exert pressure on the tissues which increases the permeability of cell membranes. This facilitates the exchange of tissue fluids between cells and vessels. Nutrients and oxygen are transported into the cells more efficiently and waste products transported out.

4 Massage speeds up venous and lymphatic drainage from the area which removes the waste products of metabolism. Following training or performance, the waste products such as lactic and pyruvic acids build up within the muscle, producing pain and stiffness. The increased pressure produced by these acids also interferes with the recovery of the muscle. Massage flushes these substances out of the muscles, thus reducing pain and stiffness and speeding up muscle recovery. Speedy recovery allows the athlete to fit in more training which will raise the standard of performance.

5 Massage increases the flexibility of the tissues. Stretching manipulations such as wringing and muscle rolling move the tissues transversely. This stretches the muscle fibres and fascial compartments to a greater extent than the longitudinal pull of stretch exercises. Muscles are also lifted and moved over supporting structures, muscle bundles are separated and fascial compartments are stretched. This greatly increases flexibility and extensibility which will improve performance and reduce the risk of injury.

6 Massage provides an early warning system to the risk of potential injury. Areas of tightness or tension may be detected in the course of a massage. Appropriate stretch manipulations and exercise can then be advised to overcome the problem and restore flexibility.

7 Massage will break down or stretch inflexible scar tissue found in muscles, tendons or ligaments of the sportsperson. These may be the result of past injuries or over-use. Scar tissue is part of the healing process and is laid down between the torn parts. It forms a tight inflexible mass which interferes with the normal function of the muscles or ligaments. Deep, short stroking movements or frictions will break down or improve the flexibility of this tissue, thus restoring function.

8 Massage will break down adhesions within the muscles. Exudate is part of the inflammatory healing process. If it is not quickly absorbed it becomes sticky and binds down the tissues, causing them to stick to one another. Deep friction will loosen and free these structures, allowing muscles and tendons to function normally.

9 Massage around joints will improve the circulation and generate warmth. This will improve the condition of joints and maintain the flexibility of joint structures. Frictions around the joint will break down adhesions from old traumas and free ligaments to function normally.

10 Massage improves flexibility and elasticity of hard, bulky, inelastic muscles following hard isometric exercise training. These exercises impede the free flow of blood to the muscle which slows down the metabolic rate. The condition of the muscle deteriorates which reduces the level of performance. Regular massage and other forms of training will prevent this deterioration.

11 Massage will promote local or general relaxation. The warmth generated in the tissues will aid relaxation. The fast removal of metabolic waste will prevent pain and stiffness developing, thus relieving tension. The rhythmic stretching manipulations promote relaxation. Slow rhythmical massage has a soothing effect on the nervous system. These movements produce a reflex response which releases tension. General massage also has an effect on the autonomic nervous system which improves relaxation.

Use of massage in sport

Massage may be used in four distinct categories to help sportspeople. Although all the basic massage manipulations may be used, certain considerations and adaptations must be made. It is important that athletes and their trainers are aware of these differences and appreciate their effects.

Massage may be given in the following instances:

- before an event or performance (pre-event massage)
- after an event or performance (post-event massage)
- as part of the training programme (training massage)
- as a rehabilitation treatment (treatment massage).

Pre-event massage

The aim of this massage is to help the body respond to the demands of increased activity and facilitate optimum performance. The objectives are:

- to increase the delivery of nutrients and oxygen to the contracting muscles
- to warm the muscles, thus improving contractility
- to improve the flexibility and extensibility of muscles
- to maintain maximum range of movement of joints.

At rest the body is in a balanced state known as homeostasis and the systems of the body must just meet the basic metabolic needs. Muscular activity requires an abundant supply of energy and the body systems must respond rapidly to meet these needs. An increased supply of nutrients and oxygen must be delivered to the working muscles. Warm-up and stretch exercises are essential prior to performance as they gradually bring the body systems up to a level which will enable the athlete to perform at maximum potential. Massage must not replace these exercises but may be used to enhance their effect.

TREATMENT TECHNIQUE

This massage must be brisk and of fairly short duration, e.g. 7–10 minutes for each area. It must be stimulating to create alertness and focus. It should concentrate on the body parts involved in the performance, but both sides of the body must be treated to maintain balance. It is usual to include the back with both upper and lower parts of the body. For example, for throwers cover the back, shoulders and arms; for runners cover the back, buttocks and legs.

A relaxing or general body massage should not be given before a performance because the athlete must remain alert and ready for action. The athlete must have experienced massage during training; s/he should not receive the first massage before performance as timing and rhythm may be affected.

Experienced therapists will develop their own massage routines and make adaptations according to the needs of the athlete. However, for the treatment to be effective, a basic routine is essential. Pre-event massage is similar to the stimulating massage described in Chapter 9. A suggested routine is as follows:

1 work towards the heart, i.e. distal to proximal with pressure upwards

2 brisk effleurage of moderate depth, progressing to greater depth

3 kneading to main muscle groups and around joints

4 wringing to main muscle groups

5 picking up to main muscle groups

6 effleurage

7 light hacking and cupping to large muscles

8 muscle rolling

9 gentle muscle shaking and compression where possible.

Finish the massage with stroking away from the heart, i.e. proximal to distal. This dilates capillaries and encourages the flow of fresh oxygenated blood into the muscles. Many therapists include passive movements of appropriate joints in the routine. This requires great care and very specific knowledge of joint movement and is not within the scope of this book.

EFFECTS

1 Massage speeds up venous drainage and produces dilation of blood vessels and capillaries. This results in more blood flow – hyperaemia which increases the availability of nutrients and oxygen required for muscle contraction.

2 Squeezing and pressure of the tissues facilitates the exchange of tissue fluids across cell membranes, increasing absorption.

3 Massage creates warmth in the tissues. Warm muscles contract more efficiently and powerfully than cold muscles, which results in better performance.

4 Warm muscles are also more flexible and extensible and are consequently less likely to tear.

5 The petrissage manipulations, such as wringing and picking up, improve the flexibility of muscle fibres and supporting fascia. This also reduces the risk of injury.

6 Massage performed around the joints warms the surrounding structures, thus increasing flexibility. This facilitates the maximum range of movement and reduces the risk of injury.

Post-event massage

The aim of this treatment is to promote speedy and complete muscle recovery and to re-establish homeostasis. The objectives are:

◆ to speed up venous and lymphatic drainage of the area and thus remove metabolic waste

◆ to increase the delivery of nutrients and oxygen to combat fatigue and aid muscle recovery

◆ to prevent or relieve pain and stiffness

◆ to relieve tension and promote relaxation

◆ to prevent tightening of fascial components and maintain flexibility

◆ to identify areas of tenderness or soreness which may indicate injury

◆ to prevent the formation of adhesions and fibrosis.

The energy for prolonged or vigorous muscle contraction is provided initially from stored adenosine triphosphate (ATP) and phosphocreatine, and then by the breakdown of glucose into pyruvic acid by a process known as glycolysis. If the body can maintain an adequate supply of oxygen (as in steady state aerobic exercises), then the pyruvic acid is completely metabolised to carbon dioxide and water. However, if the exercises are aerobic, i.e. vigorous and there is insufficient oxygen, then the pyruvic acid is converted to lactic acid which gradually builds up within the muscle. This build up of lactic acid increases the pressure within the muscle, producing pain and stiffness. It also compresses vessels and capillaries, restricting the flow of blood which reduces the availability of nutrients and oxygen, resulting in muscle fatigue and inhibiting the process of recovery.

TREATMENT TECHNIQUE

This massage should be given as soon as possible after the event and certainly within the first one to two hours. The massage will then be more effective as the waste build up is removed more quickly and the recovery will be faster. Great care must be taken when giving post-event massage as the muscles may be tender, sore and painful. This is partly due to the pressure of accumulated waste and also due to any injuries or micro-traumas which may have occurred during performance. Very light pressure should be applied initially, becoming deeper as muscle relaxation is felt. As the prime aim is to clear away metabolites, the strokes should begin proximally near the lymph nodes. This congested area is cleared first and the manipulations work downwards, gradually pushing fluids into the cleared areas (this is explained in lymph drainage in Chapter 9).

The movements begin with light stroking and effleurage, gentle muscle lifting, rolling and shaking. Kneading, wringing and picking up should not be used until the muscle has relaxed. The flesh will not be soft enough to yield to the pressure and rubbing the hard muscle will cause pain and increase tension. Changing the pressure over different areas is essential in post-event massage – it must be very light over painful, tense areas, becoming gradually deeper as the muscle is felt to relax. The therapist must develop the ability to sense the condition of the tissues through the hands and adapt the massage accordingly.

1 Begin proximally to clear the upper congested area first.

2 Gentle stroking over the part will give an indication of the condition of the tissues. This will provide feedback on areas of tension, painful spots, tightness and rigidity. Use very light movements initially.

3 Effleurage: begin proximally and work down, one hand width at a time. For example, on the leg begin on the thigh towards the inguinal nodes in the groin – push up, move down one hand width, push up, and so on until the knee is reached. Increase the depth as the muscle relaxes. Keep the movement slow and rhythmic. Then move below the knee and cover the lower leg.

4 Muscle shaking or vibrations: place the flat of the hand on the muscle and gently shake it up and down and from side to side.

5 Muscle rolling: gently grasp and lift the muscle; roll it first to one side and then to the other.

6 Work in this way until the muscles soften and then add any of the following:

◆ kneading

◆ wringing

◆ picking up.

7 Deep stroking: use the tips of the flattened fingers, the heel or the ulnar border of the hand to apply short, deep strokes to the muscle belly to separate the muscle compartments and loosen the fascia.

8 Effleurage from distal to proximal to complete the massage.

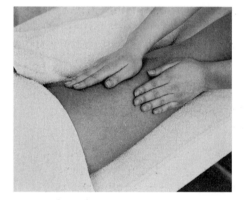

Figure 11.2 Stroking to sense condition of tissues

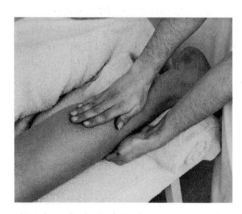

Figure 11.3 Muscle vibrations

EFFECTS

1 Massage speeds up venous and lymphatic drainage of the area. The waste product, lactic acid, is quickly removed, preventing build up within the muscle and thus reducing soreness, pain and stiffness.

2 Massage reduces the pressure and compression created by a build up of metabolic waste and produces dilation of vessels and capillaries. This increases blood flow and the delivery of nutrients and oxygen to the area, reducing muscle fatigue and aiding the recovery of the muscle. Research indicates that recovery is three to four times faster in muscles subjected to massage than in those simply allowed to rest.

3 Gentle massage warms the area and soothes sensory receptors in the skin, reducing tension and inducing relaxation.

4 Stretching manipulations such as muscle rolling, shaking and gentle wringing will maintain the flexibility of the fascia, the extensibility of muscle fibres and the movement of muscle bundles. These stretching effects are important in maintaining overall flexibility.

5 During massage experienced therapists will obtain direct feedback on the condition of the tissues. Through the hands they can sense and become aware of changes within the tissues. Pain, soreness or increased tension are highlighted. These factors may indicate minor traumas which can be immediately treated and allowed to recover, thus preventing more serious injury.

Training massage

The aim of this massage is to help the athlete achieve and maintain peak condition, thus maximising performance. This massage is very similar to post-event massage, as its main aim is to clear out the waste products and promote speedy recovery. There are, however, differences which should be noted. The objectives are:

◆ to maintain an efficient circulation and delivery of nutrients and oxygen for nourishing the tissues

◆ to quickly remove metabolic waste after a training session

◆ to promote fast recovery of the muscles, thus allowing greater frequency of training

◆ to prevent any minor injuries becoming more serious and chronic

◆ to prevent the formation of scar tissue and to stretch and break down old scar tissue

◆ to prevent the formation of adhesions and fibrosis

◆ to maintain flexibility or elasticity of muscles, fascia, tendons and ligaments

◆ to maintain and improve the range of movement at joints

◆ to relieve stress and promote relaxation.

Training massage is probably the most beneficial for the athlete. It should be given, like post-event massage, immediately following activity. This will achieve similar effects in flushing out waste products, aiding the recovery of the muscles and restoring homeostasis. Massage identifies and reduces areas of tension which could lead to serious injury. During hard training massage may be given after every session. If given every day or so, it should be fairly light. The massage should concentrate on the strained used areas, although it is important to treat both sides of the body to maintain balance. It is also important to treat antagonistic muscles equally, as increased tension in the antagonistic muscles will limit performance or leave the muscle vulnerable to injury.

Again an upper body massage including the back, or lower body massage including the back, may be given. In addition a full deep body massage should be given once a week. This reduces stress levels and promotes relaxation. This should be followed by one or two days of rest to allow recovery. A full body massage should not be given immediately before an event. At least four or five days should elapse to allow the athlete to fully recover alertness and focus.

If minor injuries occur during training, they may only become apparent during massage. If left untreated they would leave the body vulnerable to further injury. The therapist is able to identify these areas of pain or tension and treat them immediately, thus preventing more extensive or serious trauma. Many minor injuries may occur during training. The more common and easily treatable are described below.

◆ Small tears or micro-traumas may occur within muscles. These will heal with the formation of fibrous scar tissue. The extent of fibrous tissue laid down will depend on the extent of the trauma and the speed of recovery. Scar tissue forms a hard inflexible mass within the muscle which contracts over time. This reduces the extensibility and flexibility of the muscle, impairing its function. Regular massage will speed up the recovery and reduce the amount of scar tissue laid down. Massage will also maintain the suppleness of old scar tissue already present and prevent it contracting.

◆ The fascia surrounding and lying between muscles may tighten as a result of injuries or repetitive strain. This will produce pain and stiffness which will inhibit muscle action. Stretching massage will separate these fascial compartments, loosen the fascia and release the muscles to function correctly.

◆ Massage around joints will improve nourishment and maintain flexibility of joint structures. The tendons or ligaments around joints may be damaged or over-stretched (sprains) during training or performance. During the healing process, the exudate which is part of the inflammatory process may become tacky and sticky, and form adhesions which bind the tendons and ligaments to underlying structures. Frictions performed around the joint or across the tendons will help to free these structures and restore joint function.

◆ Some forms of training, such as strength training, result in bulky inflexible muscles. Massage will be very beneficial in maintaining the suppleness of these muscles. Use of isometric work, where the muscles contract but do not change in length, inhibits the flow of blood as there is no pumping action on the blood vessels. If there are insufficient rest periods, pressure is maintained on the capillary beds, further restricting blood flow, and muscle fatigue develops quickly. Massage is therefore particularly beneficial following hard isometric training.

Athletes who receive massage during the training sessions recover more quickly and can train more frequently. Many athletes suffer a high degree of stress and anxiety. A general body massage performed regularly once a week can improve the well-being of the athlete. The stress and anxiety levels are reduced, which will relieve symptoms such as headaches, irritability, listlessness and vague aches and pains, and can restore good sleep patterns.

TREATMENT TECHNIQUE

Training massage should be given regularly as part of the training schedule. It may be a full body massage or it may concentrate on the upper or lower half of the body, depending on the areas of greater stress. A half body massage will take approximately half an hour. A full body massage of up to one hour may be given once a week, provided it is not within five days or so of an event. For a half body massage begin on the side which has received most stress, but be sure to treat the other side as well. The massage can vary according to the preference of the therapist and the needs of the athlete. The following is one example of a suitable routine.

Upper body

Supine
- arm
- shoulder
- chest
- arm

Prone
- arm
- back
- upper back and shoulder
- arm

Lower body

Supine
- thigh
- lower leg
- foot
- lower leg
- thigh

Prone
- thigh
- calf
- foot
- calf
- thigh
- buttocks
- back

Use the following manipulations:

1 superficial stroking: this must be a light, sensitive exploratory movement from distal to proximal in order to introduce the massage and sense the condition of the tissues

2 effleurage: this must be light to moderate if the muscles are sore and tense, becoming deeper if the muscles relax; begin proximally

3 shaking: along the muscle to aid relaxation

4 kneading: if the muscle is soft enough

5 short stroking: to explore and release tense areas. Begin proximally (e.g. just below the groin on the thigh), use the pads of the fingers to probe upwards deeply into the tissues, move down to the next area and repeat. Cover the thigh down to the knee in this way. Where areas of tightness and tension are felt probe transversally back and forth

6 muscle rolling: lift the muscle and push from side to side from thumbs to fingers and back

7 wringing

8 double-handed pressure kneading (or thumb kneading on anterior tibials). If tightness or nodules are felt in the muscle, ease the pressure

9 shaking

10 effleurage: work down to the foot and then back up with deeper pressure.

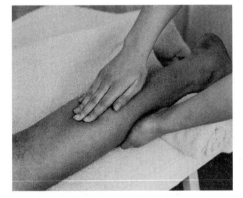

Figure 11.4 Short probing stroking

EFFECTS

1 Massage improves the circulation to the areas being worked on. The delivery of nutrients and oxygen is increased, thus improving the condition of the muscle and facilitating recovery.

2 Venous and lymphatic drainage are speeded up and metabolic waste is quickly removed from the tissues. This reduces pain and stiffness which would result from a build up of lactic acid. Recovery time is shorter and therefore more frequent training sessions may be undertaken.

3 The therapist gains feedback on the condition of the tissues during massage. Minor injuries may be quickly identified and treated, preventing more serious injuries occurring.

4 Massage reduces the formation of scar tissue following muscle tears. It also immobilises and stretches old scar tissue, improving flexibility of the muscle.

5 Massage removes the sticky exudate following injury. This in turn reduces the formation of adhesions and frees affected structures so that they function correctly.

6 Massage maintains the flexibility of fascia and fascial compartments, enabling the muscles to function efficiently.

7 Frictions around the joints will loosen and release bound ligaments, improving joint range.

8 Massage relieves pressure and rigidity within muscle groups following isometric exercise and restores muscle elasticity.

Treatment massage

The aim of this type of massage is to promote rapid healing and aid complete recovery of the tissues, thus restoring normal function. The objectives are:

◆ to reduce the inflammatory response

◆ to promote healing and reduce pain, swelling and stiffness

◆ to gradually mobilise and stretch the affected tissues

◆ to return the body to normal function.

Accurate diagnosis is crucial following injury and the athlete must be seen by a doctor as soon as possible. Those without medical training should not attempt to diagnose or treat sports injuries. However, knowing what action to take immediately before medical attention is available can reduce the extent of tissue damage. Treatment can be given by an experienced therapist if the diagnosis reveals that the injury is of a minor nature, or under the guidance of a medical practitioner.

TREATMENT TECHNIQUE

Immediate action involves:

R for rest and immobilisation to prevent further damage
I   for ice, applied immediately for vasoconstriction
C for compression to the area to reduce swelling
E for elevation, using gravity to assist drainage of exudate from the area
D for diagnosis by a doctor, on site, in a surgery or in a hospital.

REST

Rest is essential for all sudden, acute injuries because continued movement can increase the extent of the damage. Movement may increase bleeding into the tissues; it may increase the inflammatory response with increased fluid exudate and swelling of the tissues; or it may cause further tearing and damage of the muscle fibres, tendons or ligaments. Resting the part may be sufficient, but it is usually necessary to use some form of support such as splints, tubular or stocking supports, crêpe bandages, slings and collars. Care must be taken that the strapping is firm but not too tight, as this can restrict the circulation and cause further damage. The strapping must be able to stretch or give if the swelling increases.

ICE

Ice should be placed over the injured part as soon as possible. Cold will cause constriction of the blood vessels which will reduce internal bleeding and fluid exudate. This will prevent excessive bleeding and swelling. Cold also reduces the sensitivity of pain receptors and the conductivity of nerves. It numbs the area, reducing muscle spasm and tension.

Care must be taken when applying the ice as there is a risk of producing ice burns if the ice is in direct contact with the skin for some time. A wet towel should be placed on the skin to protect it and the ice placed on top. There are various ways of applying ice – freezer gel packs are the most convenient, but packs of frozen food can also be used. These are placed over the towel and held in place by another towel wrapped around the part, which will also apply compression. Ice cubes can be crushed and placed inside a towel and placed over the area. Injuries to the ankle or wrist can be treated by immersing the injured part in a bucket of iced water. The part should be held in the water for as long as is tolerable, removed for a few minutes and then re-immersed. Ice packs are kept in place for 10–15 minutes and applied every three or four hours initially, decreasing to three times a day as healing progresses.

Cold sprays are commonly used in sport as they are easy to carry and convenient to use. However, they are not as effective as ice packs as they do not cool the deeper tissues. They are effective only on superficial tissues and are not recommended for use on acute traumas. Over-use in an attempt to reach deeper tissues can result in ice burns to the skin.

COMPRESSION

Pressure applied to the area will stop the bleeding and reduce the swelling. Crêpe, tubular or stocking bandages may be used to apply pressure. A pad of cotton wool over the area, before applying the bandage, will increase the pressure over the injury. The bandage must extend above and below the injured area and may include the entire limb. The bandaging must not be too tight, as previously explained.

ELEVATION

The injured part should be supported in elevation wherever possible. Gravity will then assist the drainage of any fluid exudate away from the part. This will reduce stagnation and the formation of sticky exudate which can bind structures to each other and hamper movement.

DIAGNOSIS

Accurate diagnosis must be obtained as soon as possible,

followed by appropriate rehabilitation. This is crucial to full and complete recovery.

MASSAGE IN REHABILITATION

Massage must not be given immediately after injury as there is a risk of internal bleeding into the tissues. The treatment in the initial stages of acute injury is ice, compression and rest. Ice should be used for the first six to eight days until there is no risk of bleeding and healing is progressing. If the injuries are minor then massage may begin after two to three days. After the ice is removed the area is very gently and lightly stroked in the direction of venous return (towards the heart). If there is swelling present, the part should be elevated so that gravity can assist the drainage.

If the injuries are more serious then ice treatment is continued, but massage is not used for six to eight days until all danger of further bleeding is over and tissue healing is well under way. After six to eight days the same superficial stroking movement is used to 'sense' the condition of the tissues. As the tissues are felt to relax, deeper movements can be applied. Massage must not produce any pain or increased tension within the tissues – the pressure must be reduced or the massage stopped if this occurs. Vibrations and shaking may be used, particularly above and below the injured part.

After eight to ten days some form of heat may be used, i.e. infra-red or heat packs. This can be followed by deeper massage movements such as effleurage, kneading and muscle rolling. Heat must not be used in the initial stages of treatment as it dilates blood vessels and increases blood flow to the area. When there is no risk of bleeding and when the healing is under way, it is used to promote and hasten the healing process. Gentle heat for 10–15 minutes should be used initially, increasing to around 25 minutes. Do not overheat as this is counter-productive. Heat increases metabolic rate and promotes healing, but overheating is irritating, interferes with metabolism and slows the process of healing.

As the condition of the tissues improves, then deeper massage movements can be added to the previous regime, e.g. deep effleurage, kneading, wringing (to stretch muscle fibres and fascia), muscle rolling (to maintain flexibility), short deep probing stroking (to stretch fibrous tissue), frictions into tight areas (to stretch any adhesions), deep effleurage and light stroking. These movements must only be used if there is no pain. Return to gentle stroking if any pain or tension is evoked by other movements.

Athletes must allow time for full recovery following trauma and must build up the training routine very gradually. If they return too soon or train too hard, serious chronic conditions, which will permanently affect performance, may result.

Contra-indications to sports massage

- infections or contagious skin diseases
- open wounds or abrasions
- internal bleeding or haemorrhage, or any potential risk of bleeding
- broken bones
- severe or extensive bruising
- muscle ruptures
- tendon or ligament ruptures
- burns
- thrombosis or phlebitis
- bursitis
- arthritis
- undiagnosed areas of deep pain
- tumours

?

1 Explain six benefits of massage to a sports-person.

2 Give the four categories where massage would be used.

3 Explain briefly why hard training must be balanced with adequate rest.

4 List any six symptoms which may result from over-training and incomplete rest.

5 Explain what is meant by the term 'homeostasis'.

6 List the objectives of:

   (a) pre-event massage

   (b) post-event massage.

7 Explain the effects of pre-event massage.

8 Explain briefly why lactic acid builds up within a muscle during exercise and how massage helps its removal.

9 Suggest the manipulations you would use for a post-event massage. Give reasons for your selection.

10 Explain why training massage helps the athlete to train more frequently.

11 List six common minor injuries that may occur during training or performance.

12 Give the immediate first aid procedure following injury.

13 Explain why massage should not be given immediately following injury.

Index

···